It's easy to get lost in the cancer world

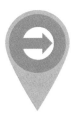

Let NCCN Guidelines for Patients® be your guide

✓ Step-by-step guides to the cancer care options likely to have the best results

✓ Based on treatment guidelines used by health care providers worldwide

✓ Designed to help you discuss cancer treatment with your doctors

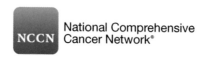

NCCN Guidelines for Patients® are developed by the National Comprehensive Cancer Network® (NCCN®)

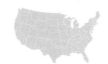

NCCN

✓ An alliance of leading cancer centers across the United States devoted to patient care, research, and education

Cancer centers that are part of NCCN:
NCCN.org/cancercenters

NCCN Clinical Practice Guidelines in Oncology (NCCN Guidelines®)

✓ Developed by experts from NCCN cancer centers using the latest research and years of experience

✓ For providers of cancer care all over the world

✓ Expert recommendations for cancer screening, diagnosis, and treatment

Free online at
NCCN.org/guidelines

NCCN Guidelines for Patients

✓ Present information from the NCCN Guidelines in an easy-to-learn format

✓ For people with cancer and those who support them

✓ Explain the cancer care options likely to have the best results

Free online at
NCCN.org/patientguidelines

These NCCN Guidelines for Patients are based on the NCCN Guidelines® for Non-Small Cell Lung Cancer, Version 3.2022 – March 16, 2022.

NCCN Foundation seeks to support the millions of patients and their families affected by a cancer diagnosis by funding and distributing NCCN Guidelines for Patients. NCCN Foundation is also committed to advancing cancer treatment by funding the nation's promising doctors at the center of innovation in cancer research. For more details and the full library of patient and caregiver resources, visit NCCN.org/patients.

National Comprehensive Cancer Network (NCCN) / NCCN Foundation
3025 Chemical Road, Suite 100
Plymouth Meeting, PA 19462
215.690.0300

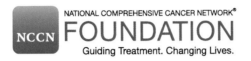

NCCN Guidelines for Patients are supported by funding from the NCCN Foundation®

To make a gift or learn more, please visit NCCNFoundation.org/donate
or e-mail PatientGuidelines@NCCN.org.

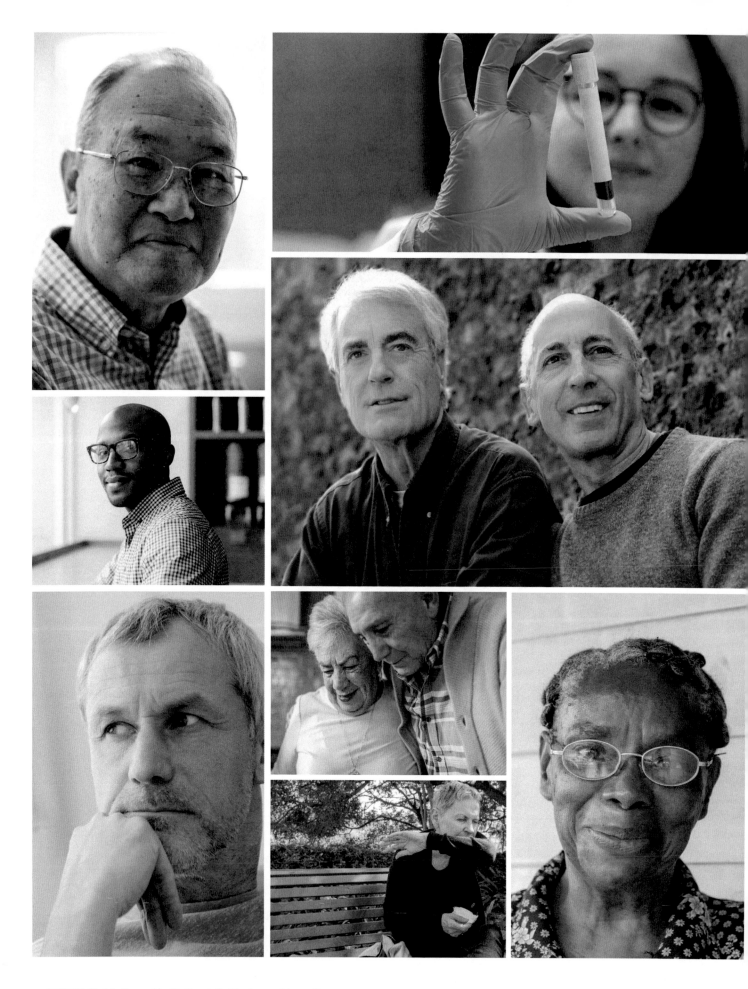

NCCN Guidelines for Patients®: Early and Locally
Advanced Non-Small Cell Lung Cancer, 2022   4

Contents

1
Lung cancer basics

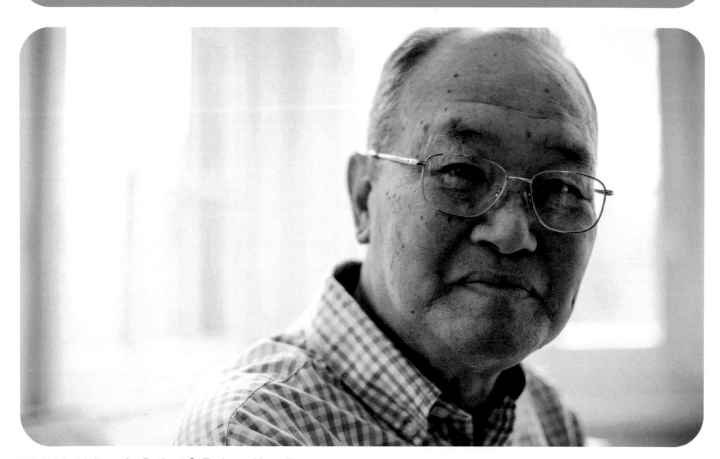

Lung cancer starts in the cells of the lungs. Non-small cell lung cancer is the most common type of lung cancer. This chapter answers some common questions about this cancer when it is early or locally advanced.

What is lung cancer?

Lung cancer is a cancer of lung cells. Other cancers that have spread to the lungs are not lung cancers. For example, stomach cancer that has spread to the lungs is still stomach cancer.

The lungs are the main organs of the respiratory system. They deliver oxygen to the blood and remove carbon dioxide from the blood.

Lung cancer often forms from cells that line the airways

Almost all lung cancers are carcinomas. Lung carcinomas form from cells that line the airways of the lungs. The airways of the lungs are called the bronchus, bronchioli, and alveoli.

Lung carcinomas are divided into 2 main groups based on how the cells look.

> Small cell lung cancer (SCLC) is a cancer of neuroendocrine cells. The NCCN Guidelines for Patients® on SCLC can be found at NCCN.org/ patientguidelines.

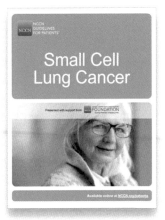

> Non-small cell lung cancer (NSCLC) is much more common than SCLC.

Airways of the lungs

The air you breathe moves through a series of airways. It travels down your throat and through your windpipe (trachea). The windpipe splits into 2 airways called bronchi. Inside the lung, each bronchus branches off into the parts of the lung, called lobes. The right lung has 3 lobes, and the left lung has 2 lobes. The bronchi divide into smaller airways called the bronchioli. At the end of the bronchioli are sacs called alveoli. Oxygen is transferred from air into the blood in the alveoli.

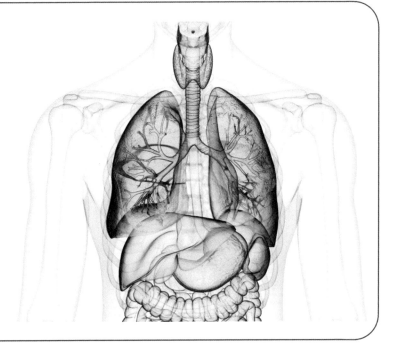

There are several types of NSCLC

Each type of NSCLC forms from a particular kind of cell. Below are common types of NSCLC:

> Adenocarcinoma often forms from cells that line the alveoli and make mucus. It is the most common type of lung cancer.

> Large cell carcinoma forms from any of the large cells that are found throughout the airways.

> Squamous cell carcinoma forms from cells that line the bronchi.

What are the stages of lung cancer?

The stage of lung cancer describes the extent of the cancer in the body. It is used to assess the outlook of the cancer called the prognosis. It is used to plan treatment. It is also used for research.

For some people, cancer staging is done twice. The stage assigned before any tissue (biopsy) testing is called the clinical stage. The second stage is called the pathologic stage and is based on tissue tests. Cancer that is outside of the lungs may not be found until after surgery.

Staging is based on the AJCC system

The American Joint Committee on Cancer (AJCC) staging manual is used to stage lung cancer. The stages of NSCLC range from stage 0 to stage 4. Often, the stages are written with Roman numerals—stages 0, I, II, III, and IV.

What is cancer?

Cancer is a disease that affects cell growth. When cells become cancerous, they don't behave like normal cells. They break the rules of normal cell growth.

• Lung cancer cells make many new cancer cells. They also do not die when they should. This overgrowth of cancer cells becomes a mass of tissue called a tumor.

• Lung cancer cells don't stay in place. They can grow through the airway and into the lung tissue. They can grow through the lung wall and invade other body parts.

• Lung cancer cells can break away from a tumor and spread. They can enter the bloodstream or a fluid called lymph and spread to other places.

This out-of-control cell growth can harm the body. Cancer cells crowd out and overpower normal cells. Without enough normal cells, cancer cells can cause organs to stop working.

Scientists have learned a great deal about cancer. As a result, today's treatments work better than treatments in the past. Also, many people with cancer have more than one treatment option.

Stage 0 cancer is only in the airway

Stage 0 is rare. Abnormal or cancer cells have formed in the airways but haven't grown into the lung tissue. Stage 0 is also called carcinoma in situ.

Stage 1 through 3 cancers haven't spread far at the time of diagnosis

Stage 1, stage 2, and stage 3 cancers have grown into lung tissue. Some have spread to nearby disease-fighting tissue called lymph nodes.

Stage 4 cancer has spread far

To be stage 4, lung cancer must have already spread far by the time of diagnosis. Most lung cancers are stage 4 at diagnosis. Lung cancer tends to spread to these body parts:

> Brain, liver, bone, and adrenal glands

> From one lung to the other lung

DO NOT be afraid to ask your medical team ANY questions at any time!!! Your questions will help you and them. No question is stupid."

– Steve
  Cancer survivor

What stages are early and locally advanced lung cancers?

Stage 1 and stage 2 cancers are also described as early-stage cancers. Stage 3 cancers are locally advanced.

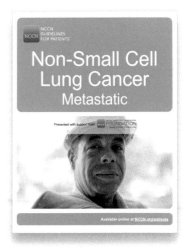

Some early and locally advanced cancers spread far after diagnosis and then are called metastatic cancer. Learn about treatment of metastatic cancers, including stage 4, in *NCCN Guidelines for Patients: Metastatic Non-Small Cell Lung Cancer*, available at NCCN.org/patientguidelines.

What are the symptoms of early and locally advanced lung cancer?

Early cancers may not cause symptoms but many advanced cancers do. Some symptoms of lung cancer are:

> A new cough that doesn't go away

> A chronic cough that worsens

> Coughing up bloody mucus

> Getting short of breath quicker than before

> Ongoing pain in the chest or upper back

> Frequent lung infections that don't go away or keep coming back

Lung cancer is often found because of symptoms and less often found in x-rays before symptoms start. Lung cancers may be found by chance in x-rays or through a cancer screening program. Learn more about screening in *NCCN Guidelines for Patients: Lung Cancer Screening*, available at NCCN.org/patientguidelines.

Can early and locally advanced lung cancer be treated?

Yes! For most lung cancers, the aim of treatment is to reduce symptoms, control the cancer, and extend life. Newer treatments are better at controlling the cancer and improving quality of life.

At this time, few lung cancers are cured. Early-stage cancers are highly treatable and sometimes curable. Locally advanced cancers are rarely cured. A cure may be possible if the cancer didn't spread much.

Treatment takes team work

A team of health care providers is involved in diagnosing and treating lung cancers. Your primary doctor may be the first to suspect you have lung cancer and refer you to specialists. The diagnostic, treatment, and supportive care experts are explained throughout this book. These experts are supported by nurses, technicians, and assistants, who are often on the frontline of cancer care. Patient navigators can help you through the maze of cancer care.

Key points

> Lung cancer is a cancer of lung cells. Other cancers that spread to the lungs are not lung cancer.

> Lung cancer often starts in the cells that line the airways. These cancers are called carcinomas. Non-small cell lung cancer (NSCLC) is a group of carcinomas.

> Common types of NSCLC are adenocarcinoma, squamous cell carcinoma, and large cell carcinoma.

> The cancer stage is a rating of the extent of the cancer. Stages of lung cancer range from stage 0 to stage 4.

> Stage 1, stage 2, and stage 3 cancers have not spread far from the lung tumor.

> Early cancers often do not cause symptoms but many advanced cancers do.

> A team of experts will work together and with you to diagnose and treat the cancer as well as support you.

2
Lung nodules

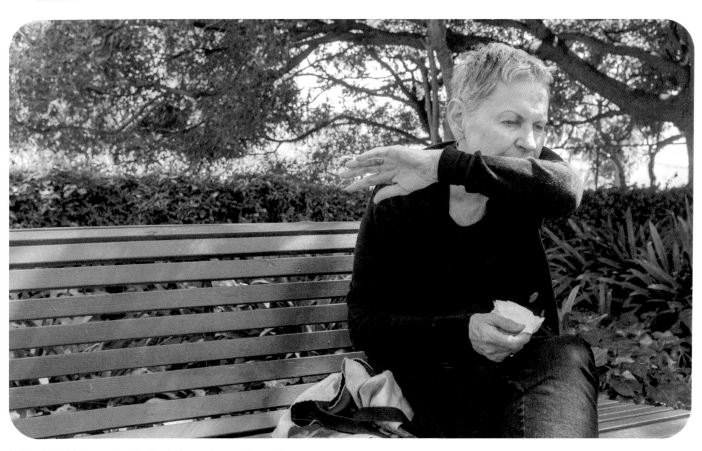

Many people have small masses of tissue in their lungs. These small masses are called nodules. A nodule may have been found in your lung by chance. This chapter discusses how doctors decide if this nodule is cancer.

Lung nodule experts

There are very few nerves inside the lungs. Without nearby nerves, nodules don't cause symptoms. They are often found by chance on x-rays for an unrelated health problem. On x-rays, nodules may be called spots or shadows.

Nodules can be caused by cancer, infections, scar tissue, and other health conditions. Most nodules are not cancer but some are. It takes a team of experts to decide if a nodule is cancer. Your team should include the following board-certified experts:

> A **pulmonologist** is a doctor who's an expert of lung diseases.

> A **thoracic radiologist** is a doctor who's an expert of imaging of the chest. Imaging makes pictures of the insides of the body.

> A **thoracic surgeon** is a doctor who's an expert in operations within the chest.

To decide if a nodule is cancer, your team will do the following:

> Assess your risk for lung cancer

> Review images and order more imaging if there may be cancer

> Perform a procedure called a biopsy if needed

At risk for lung cancer

Anyone can get lung cancer, but some people are more at risk. A risk factor is anything that increases your chance of lung cancer. Risk factors for lung cancer are listed in Guide 1.

Some people with many risk factors never get lung cancer. Some people with no risk factors do get lung cancer. Doctors are still learning why one person gets lung cancer and another does not.

Tobacco smoke
The biggest risk factor for lung cancer is smoking tobacco. There are more than 50 compounds in tobacco smoke known to cause cancer. Any smoking increases your risk of lung cancer. The more and longer you smoke, the higher your risk.

If you quit smoking, your risk for lung cancer will go down somewhat. Ask your health care providers for help to quit.

Guide 1 Risk factors for lung cancer
Current or past smoking
Advanced age
Certain cancers and cancer treatments
Family history of lung cancer
Exposure to cancer-causing agents
COPD or pulmonary fibrosis

Researchers are studying ways to prevent lung cancer caused by smoking. Treatments to prevent cancer are called chemopreventive agents. Ask your health care providers if there is a clinical trial on preventing lung cancer that you could join.

Secondhand smoke is the fumes from tobacco smoked by others. The risk of lung cancer increases as the exposure to second-hand smoke increases.

Age
As you age, you are more likely to get cancer. In recent years, half of the people who were diagnosed with lung cancer were over 71 years of age. Only 7 out of 100 people with lung cancer were under the age of 55 years.

Cancer and cancer treatment
The risk for lung cancer increases after having some types of cancer:

> Having had lung cancer increases your risk for other lung cancers.

> If you had lymphoma, you are more likely to get lung cancer.

> If you've had another smoking-related cancer, such as head and neck cancer, your risk for lung cancer is increased.

Some cancer treatments also increase the risk of lung cancer:

> The risk increases after receiving radiation therapy in the chest, especially if you smoke.

> Treatment of Hodgkin lymphoma with an alkylating cancer drug increases the risk of lung cancer too.

Family history of lung cancer
Your risk for lung cancer is increased if your parent, sibling, or child has had lung cancer. Your risk is even higher if the lung cancer occurred at a young age or among multiple relatives.

Cancer-causing agents
There are several agents known to cause lung cancer. You are more likely to get lung cancer after exposure to these agents:

> Radon

> Asbestos

> Arsenic, beryllium, cadmium, chromium, nickel (metallic metals)

> Coal smoke, soot, silica, diesel fumes

Exposure to these agents may happen at work or home. The risk after exposure is higher for people who also smoke.

Other lung diseases
Two lung diseases have been linked to lung cancer.

> Chronic obstructive pulmonary disease (COPD) makes breathing hard because the lung tissue is damaged or there's too much mucus.

> Pulmonary fibrosis is major scarring of lung tissue that makes it hard to breathe.

Signs of cancer on imaging

Lung nodules may be first detected by chest x-rays (CXR), computed tomography (CT), or positron emission tomography (PET) scans. Your radiologist will review the images to decide if the nodule may be cancer. Important test results are the features of the nodule, abnormal lung tissue, and PET hot spots.

Features of the nodule

Nodules caused by cancer have specific features. First, they aren't likely to have calcium. Second, they often have rough edges and odd shapes. Other very important features are the nodule size and density.

> Nodules with cancer often grow faster and are larger than ones without cancer.

> Nodules with cancer are most often solid or part solid.

Solid nodules are dense. They look like a thick cloud on imaging. Non-solid nodules are less dense than solid nodules. They look like a hazy cloud on imaging. Non-solid nodules are also called ground-glass opacities (GGOs) or ground-glass nodules (GGNs). Part-solid nodules have both high and low areas of density.

Abnormal lung tissue

Besides nodules, imaging may show other abnormal findings. It may show tissue inflammation, tissue scarring, or both.

PET hot spots

PET shows how your cells are using a simple form of sugar called glucose. To create the pictures, a sugar radiotracer is put into your body. The radiotracer emits a small amount of energy that is detected by the imaging machine.

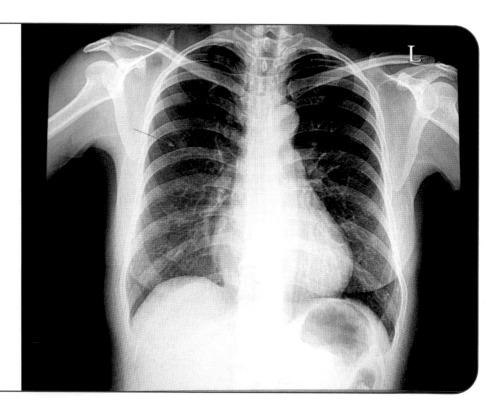

Lung nodule

A lung nodule is a small mass of tissue in the lung. Many people have lung nodules. Most are not cancer. When nodules are found by imaging, you may receive more scans to assess if the nodule is cancer.

Cancer quickly uses glucose so it appears "hot" in images. The more sugar the cancer cells use, the quicker they are growing. Other health problems can cause hot spots, too. Cancer detected by PET often needs to be confirmed with other testing.

Follow-up care of nodules

Your team will check on nodules that may be cancer. The type of follow-up you will receive is based on nodule features, such as density and size.

Solid nodules

Your team will consider your risk for lung cancer and the nodule size to plan the next step of care. Your risk is low if you have minor or no risk factors. You must not have smoked or smoked very little. Follow-up care of solid nodules found by chance is listed in Guide 2.

Part-solid and non-solid nodules

The next steps of care are based on the number and size of nodules. Many of these nodules go away in time without treatment. Those that remain are not likely to become

Guide 2
Follow-up care of solid nodules

Low risk for lung cancer	Nodule is smaller than 6 mm	No routine imaging is needed
	Nodule is between 6 and 8 mm	Get a CT scan 6 to 12 months after the first scan of the nodule. If there is no increase in nodule size or density, your doctor may order another CT scan 18 to 24 months after the first scan.
	Nodule is larger than 8 mm	• Your doctor may order CT in 3 months • Your doctor may order PET/CT now • Your doctor may order a biopsy now
High risk of lung cancer	Nodule is smaller than 6 mm	It is an option to get a CT scan at 12 months after the first scan of the nodule. If there is no increase in nodule size or density, no routine imaging is needed.
	Nodule is between 6 and 8 mm	Get a CT scan 6 to 12 months after the first scan of the nodule. If there is no increase in nodule size or density, your doctor may order another CT scan 18 to 24 months after the first scan.
	Nodule is larger than 8 mm	• Your doctor may order CT in 3 months • Your doctor may order PET/CT now • Your doctor may order a biopsy now

a problem. Follow-up care for part-solid and non-solid nodules found by chance is listed in Guide 3.

Nodules are measured in millimeters (mm). The tip of a crayon is about 2 mm.

Why is another CT needed? Often, one CT scan doesn't clearly show whether the nodule is cancer. Instead, CT needs to be repeated over time. Low-dose CT (LDCT) or a diagnostic CT may be used.

LDCT uses much less radiation than a standard scan. It also does not require contrast. Contrast is a substance that is injected into the body to make clearer pictures. LDCT is preferred by NCCN experts for cancer screening unless a clearer picture is needed.

Your radiologist will compare the first (baseline) CT with follow-up CT scans. Signs of cancer include increases in nodule size or density. If the nodule is likely cancer, read Chapter 3 next.

Guide 3
Follow-up care of part-solid and non-solid nodules

1 part-solid nodule	**Nodule is smaller than 6 mm**	No routine imaging is needed
	Nodule is 6 mm or larger	Get a CT scan in 3 to 6 months after the first scan of the nodule. If there's no nodule growth and the solid part remains smaller than 6 mm, repeat CT every year for 5 years. If the solid part is 6 mm or larger, your doctor may order PET/CT or a biopsy.
1 non-solid nodule	**Nodule is smaller than 6 mm**	No routine imaging is needed
	Nodule 6 mm or larger	Get a CT scan in 6 to 12 months after the first scan of the nodule. If there is no increase in nodule size or density, repeat CT every 2 years until 5 years after the first scan.
2 or more non-solid or part-solid nodules	**Nodules are smaller than 6 mm**	Get a CT scan in 3 to 6 months after the first scan of the nodule. If there is no increase in nodule size or density, your doctor may order another CT at 2 and 4 years after the first scan.
	Nodules are 6 mm or larger	Get a CT scan in 3 to 6 months after the first scan of the nodule. The next steps depend on the nodule that is the most likely to be cancer.

Why get a PET/CT scan? CT combined with PET may find cancer quicker than repeated CT scans. PET/CT is also useful for showing signs of cancer spreading in the body.

Your whole body will be scanned or the scan will extend from your neck to your knees. If the nodule is likely cancer, read Chapter 3 next.

Why get a biopsy? If your doctor strongly suspects cancer, a biopsy may save time by allowing you to start treatment earlier. A biopsy is a procedure that removes tissue or fluid for testing. Read Chapter 3 to learn more about biopsies.

There are reasons not to get a biopsy:

- It may be better to wait and repeat CT.

- A biopsy may not be needed before treatment of early cancers.

- Sometimes, a biopsy can't be done.

Keep seeking out information and read information again as the diagnosis and treatment process continues.

– Lung cancer survivor

Key points

- It takes a team of experts to assess lung nodules for cancer.

- Tobacco smoking is the biggest risk factor for lung cancer.

- Signs of cancer can be found with imaging. For lung cancer, doctors assess a nodule's features, the condition of the lung tissue, and for PET hot spots.

- Doctors assess changes in a nodule with a series of CT scans. Nodules that quickly increase in size or density are more likely to be cancer.

- Tissue from the nodule may be sampled by a procedure called a biopsy and tested for cancer.

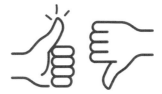

Let us know what you think!

Please take a moment to complete an online survey about the NCCN Guidelines for Patients.

NCCN.org/patients/response

3
Initial tests for lung cancer

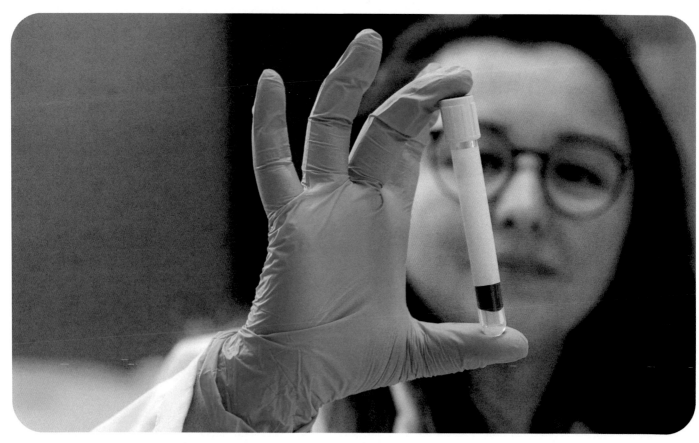

If your doctor suspects that you have lung cancer, several tests are needed. It is important to get the right tests to learn about the cancer and your health.

Goals of testing

When lung cancer is suspected, you will need to have several tests. These tests are needed to:

> Diagnose—identify the illness, and if there is cancer, identify the cell type

> Stage the cancer by testing areas to which the cancer may have spread

> Assess your general health and well-being

This chapter explains the first tests that you may get, so your cancer care team can do a complete workup. Your team will review the test results and assess what are your treatment options. Talk with your team about your options and decide together what treatment plan is best for you.

This chapter also explains some specialized services that you'll receive. It's important to start to receive these services right after a lung cancer diagnosis. They can improve your quality of life and may also help you live longer.

Tips for testing

Results from blood tests, imaging, and biopsies will be used to decide your treatment plan. It's important you understand what these tests mean. Ask questions and keep copies of your test results. Online patient portals are a handy way to access your test results.

Remember these tips for testing:

- Bring someone with you to doctor visits, if possible.

- Write down questions and take notes during appointments. Don't be afraid to ask your care team questions. Get to know your care team and help them get to know you.

- Get copies of blood tests, imaging results, and reports about the specific type of cancer you have.

- Organize your papers. Create files for insurance forms, medical records, and test results. You can do the same on your computer.

- Keep a list of contact information for everyone on your care team. Add it to your phone. Hang the list on your refrigerator or keep it in a place where someone can access it in an emergency. Keep your primary care provider informed of any changes.

Health history and exam

A standard part of a cancer evaluation is a health history and exam. These tests and others that are used to assess early and locally advanced lung cancer are listed in Guide 4.

Medical history

Expect your doctor to review your health in detail. This is known as taking a medical history. Your doctor will want to know a lot about your past and current health. You will likely be asked about:

> Illnesses and injuries

> Symptoms like unexplained weight loss, trouble breathing, chest pain, and cough

> Prescribed and over-the-counter medicines, herbs, and supplements

Smoking history

You can get lung cancer even if you never smoked. If you have lungs, you can get lung cancer. But, smoking does increase your chance of getting lung cancer.

Tell your doctors if you smoke or have smoked in the past. Smoking is often measured by packs per day and the number of years that you have smoked.

Family history

Be prepared to discuss the health problems of your close blood relatives. Such family members include brothers, sisters, parents, and grandparents. Some cancers and other health conditions can run in families.

Guide 4
Initial tests and services for early and locally advanced lung cancer

Health history and exam	• Medical history including weight loss and smoking history • Physical exam and performance status
Blood tests	• CBC with differential • Chemistry profile
Imaging	• Diagnostic CT of the chest and upper abdomen • FDG PET/CT
Cancer cell tests	• Biopsy or surgery to remove tissue samples • Pathology review to assess for lung cancer
Services	• Smoking treatment • Supportive care

Physical exam

Your doctor will also perform a thorough physical exam of your body. This exam may include:

> Checking your vital signs—blood pressure, heart rate, breathing rate, and body temperature—and assessing your overall appearance

> Feeling and listening to organs, including your spleen and liver

> Feeling for enlarged lymph nodes, which are small clusters of disease-fighting tissue

> Assessing your level of pain, if any, when you are touched

Physical ability

Based on your history and exam, your doctor will rate your performance status. Performance status is your ability to do day-to-day activities. Doctors use it to assess if you can undergo certain treatments.

Blood tests

Blood tests can measure blood cells, proteins, and chemicals in the bloodstream. They are commonly used to screen for disease. They are also used to assess if cancer is affecting organs.

Samples of your blood will be removed with a needle that is inserted into a vein. This is called a blood draw. You may need to fast from food and most liquids for hours before the draw.

CBC with differential

If not done recently, a complete blood count (CBC) with differential is needed.

> A CBC measures parts of the blood including counts of white blood cells, red blood cells, and platelets.

> A differential measures the counts of the most common types of white blood cells—basophils, neutrophils, eosinophils, monocytes, and lymphocytes. It also checks if the cell counts are in balance with each other.

Chemistry profile

Chemicals in your blood come from your liver, bone, and other organs. A chemistry profile assesses if the chemicals in your blood are too low or high.

Imaging

Imaging makes pictures of the insides of your body. It can show cancer in deep tissue, lymph nodes, or distant body parts. A radiologist is a doctor who's an expert in reading images. This doctor will convey the test results to your other doctors.

Diagnostic computed tomography (CT) is often the first scan done to stage the cancer. You will also need a PET/CT scan. PET is short for positron emission tomography.

Your doctors will use these scans to plan where to biopsy and which treatment is best. Scans that were done more than 60 days ago should not be used to decide your treatment. Some people need more imaging, like a brain scan, which is discussed in Chapter 4.

Diagnostic CT

CT makes a more detailed image than a plain x-ray. It takes many pictures of your body from different angles using x-rays. A computer then combines the pictures to make a 3-D image.

A diagnostic CT involves a higher dose of radiation and contrast. Contrast is a substance that is often injected into the bloodstream. It makes the images easier to read. For cancer staging, images of your chest and upper abdomen are needed.

FDG PET/CT

A PET/CT scan may detect cancer that was not found by CT alone. PET detects cancer with a radioactive sugar and special camera. The radioactive sugar, called fluorodeoxyglucose (FDG), will be injected into your vein.

Cancer quickly uses sugar so it appears "hot" in images. Other health problems can cause hot spots, too. Cancer detected by PET/CT often needs to be confirmed with biopsy or other imaging.

Cancer tests

To diagnose lung cancer, bits of tissue need to be removed for testing. Your team will choose a method that removes tissue that likely has cancer. Your team will also consider the risk and ease of methods and what method you prefer.

Your team may try to diagnose and stage the cancer at the same time. The body part that likely has cancer and is farthest from the lung tumor will be sampled and tested.

A biopsy or surgery is used to remove tissue for testing

> **External needle biopsies** involve guiding a thin needle through your skin and into the tumor. These procedures include transthoracic needle aspiration (TTNA), core needle biopsies, pericardiocentesis, and thoracentesis.

> **Down-the-throat biopsies** involve guiding tools down your throat into your windpipe or esophagus. These procedures include standard bronchoscopy, navigational bronchoscopy, radial endobronchial ultrasound (EBUS) bronchoscopy, endoscopic ultrasound (EUS)-guided biopsies, and robotic bronchoscopy.

> **Portal surgeries** involve making small openings (ports) into your chest. Small tools are inserted through the ports to remove tissue. Compared to open surgery, this technique is "minimally invasive." These surgeries include mediastinoscopy and thoracoscopy. Thoracoscopy is also called video-assisted thoracoscopic surgery (VATS).

> **Open surgery** involves making a large cut through your chest wall to remove tissue. You may have open surgery when other methods won't work or a larger piece of tissue is needed.

Tissue samples may be removed before or at the time of treatment

Some people can wait to be diagnosed until the day of surgical treatment. If a nodule is very likely to be cancer, a biopsy done in advance would increase health risks, time spent, and costs. Instead, a biopsy or surgery can be done right before surgical treatment. More lung tissue may be removed if the diagnosis is cancer.

There are times when it is better to diagnose before treatment:

> You shouldn't wait until treatment if your doctors strongly suspect a cancer other than lung cancer.

> An early diagnosis is also needed before treatments called radiation therapy and chemoradiation.

> If you're having surgery, it may be too hard or risky to diagnose on the same day as treatment.

The removed tissue must be large enough for testing

The tissue must be large enough to run several special lab tests. At some cancer centers, the pathologist checks the tissue size right after removal. This method is called rapid on-site evaluation (ROSE). It helps to prevent having the same procedure a second time.

Making a plan to remove tissue

It takes a team to decide the best steps to remove tissue. Removing tissue for cancer testing is not always easy. Your team should include doctors who work a lot with people who have cancer:

- Thoracic radiologist

- Interventional radiologist

- Thoracic surgeon

- Pulmonologist

When planning, doctors think about the size and location of tumors, your health history, and their experience. They rely on the results of the physical exam and imaging.

The plan to diagnose and stage lung cancer differs between people. A plan that is best for you may not be the best plan for another person. Your doctors will form a plan for you based on decisions to:

- Diagnose and stage at the same time or separately

- Sample tissue by biopsy or surgery

- Diagnose before or at the time of surgical treatment

A pathologist will assess for cancer

Tissue removed during biopsy or surgery is sent to a doctor called a pathologist. Pathologists are experts in tissue and cells and diagnosing cancer. In a lab, a pathologist will look at the tissue with a microscope. The pathologist will preserve remaining tissue for possible future testing.

The pathologist will study the tumor to classify the disease. This is called histologic typing. The pathology report will state if the cancer started in the lung or elsewhere. If the cancer started in the lung, the report will also list the type of lung cancer. Cell (histologic) types of lung cancer include:

> Squamous cell carcinoma

> Adenocarcinoma

> Large-cell lung carcinoma

> Small cell carcinoma

> Mixed and rare types

Your pathology report

Lab results used for diagnosis are put into a pathology report. This report will be sent to your doctor. It's used to plan your treatment.

Ask for a copy of the report. Ask your doctor to review your results with you. Take notes and ask questions.

Lung biopsy

A biopsy removes tissue or fluid from the body for testing. There are many types of biopsies for lung tumors. Your doctors will plan a biopsy that removes enough tissue and has the least impact on you.

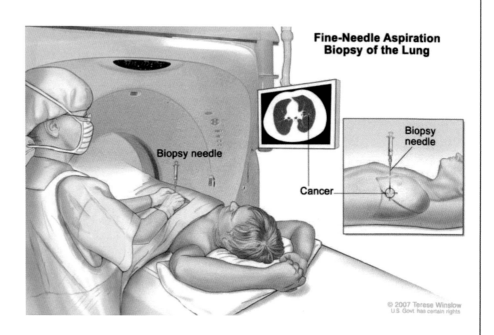

Fine-Needle Aspiration Biopsy of the Lung

Biopsy needle

Biopsy needle

Cancer

© 2007 Terese Winslow
U.S. Govt. has certain rights

Services after cancer diagnosis

Start supportive care early

Supportive care aims to improve your quality of life. It is also sometimes called palliative care. Supportive care is important for everyone, not just people at the end of life. In fact, it has been shown to extend and enhance life for people with lung cancer.

Supportive care can address many needs. It includes care for health problems caused by cancer or cancer treatment. You can get help with making treatment decisions. You can get help with coordination of care between health providers.

Your palliative care doctor will work with your oncologists to provide you the best care. Other specialists who may be involved in your care include:

> Respiratory therapists

> Rehabilitation specialists

> Registered dietitians

> Social workers

It's never too late to quit smoking

If you smoke, it is important to quit. Smoking can limit how well cancer treatment works.

Nicotine addiction is one of the hardest addictions to stop. The stress of having cancer may make it harder to quit.

There is help. Ask your health care providers about counseling and drugs to help you quit.

If you tried to quit before, try again. Most people slip or relapse before quitting for good.

Key points

> If your doctors suspect you have cancer, you'll undergo a series of tests and exams.

> Be ready to tell your doctors about any health problems and treatments you've had in your lifetime.

> Your doctors will examine your body for signs of disease. The exam will include touching parts of your body to see if anything feels abnormal.

> Your doctors will rate your ability to do day-to-day activities in order to decide your treatment options.

> Your doctors will order blood tests. Blood tests are used to look for signs of cancer.

> Diagnostic CT can help show where the cancer has spread. PET/CT may detect cancer that CT did not.

> A biopsy or surgery is needed to remove tissue samples for cancer testing. Doctors use imaging to decide what tissue should be removed and how best to remove it. If you will undergo surgery, a diagnosis of lung cancer may be deferred until the day of treatment.

> A pathologist will study the removed tissue with a microscope. If there is cancer, the pathologist will identify the type of cell from which the cancer formed.

> Supportive care aims to improve your quality of life. It is important for everyone, not just people at the end of life.

> Ask your doctor for help to quit smoking. Quitting may improve treatment results.

4
Treatment by cancer stage

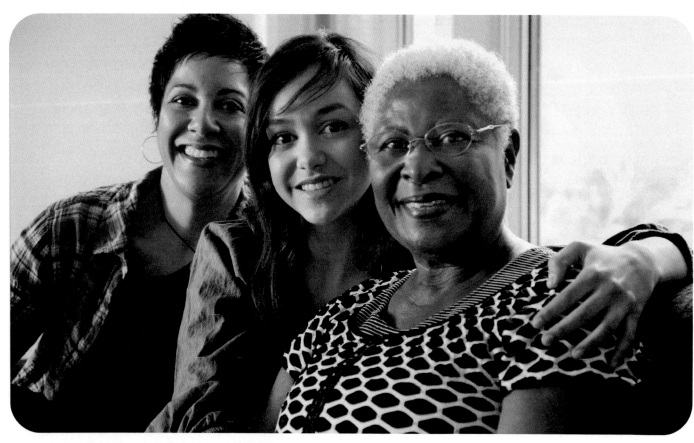

A cancer stage is a rating of the growth and spread of cancer. It is an important factor in treatment planning. Read this chapter to learn more about staging and how it is used to plan treatment.

TNM staging system

The American Joint Committee on Cancer (AJCC) staging manual is used to stage lung cancer. In this manual, a TNM system is used to score different areas of cancer growth. Your doctors will assign a score to each letter. These scores will be combined to assign the cancer a stage.

T = Tumor

The T score describes the primary tumor. The primary tumor is the main group of cancer cells in the lung. The T scores are based on:

> The size of the primary tumor measured in centimeters (cm)

> Invasive growth of the primary tumor into nearby body parts, such as the chest wall

> The number of tumors in a lung

There are several T scores. Each score has a number that stands for a level of tumor growth. The more serious the growth, the higher the T score. See Guide 5 for a brief description of T scores used for treatment planning in this book.

Guide 5 T scores	
T1	A T1 tumor is 3 cm or smaller.
T2a	A T2a tumor is larger than 3 cm but no larger than 4 cm. It may have grown into the inner lining of the lung or the main airway. It may have caused the lung to collapse or swell.
T2b	A T2b tumor is larger than 4 cm but no larger than 5 cm. It may have grown into the inner lining of the lung or the main airway. It may have caused the lung to collapse or inflame.
T3	A T3 tumor may have one or more of these features: • Tumor size is larger than 5 cm but no larger than 7 cm. • Invasion into the chest wall, phrenic nerve, outer lining of the lung, or heart's lining. • Multiple related tumors in same lobe of the lung.
T4	A T4 tumor may have one or more of these features: • Tumor size is larger than 7 cm. • Invasion into the diaphragm, middle of the chest, heart or its major blood vessels, windpipe or the area below, nerve to the voicebox, esophagus, or spine. • Related tumors in more than 1 lobe of the lung.

N = Nodes

The N score describes cancer growth in nearby lymph nodes. Lymph nodes are small, oval-shaped structures that help fight disease. The N score is based on:

> The spread of cancer to lymph nodes in the lung.

> The spread of cancer to lymph nodes just outside the lung.

> The spread of cancer to lymph nodes far from the lung.

There are several N scores. Each score has a number for the level of cancer spread in lymph nodes. The more serious the spread, the higher the N score. See Guide 6 for a brief description of N scores used for treatment planning in this book.

M = Metastasis

The M score tells you if the cancer has spread far from the lung. The spread of cancer is called metastasis. Lung cancer tends to travel to the brain, the adrenal glands, and from one lung to the other. M0 means the cancer has not spread far. There are three M1 scores:

> M1a means the cancer has spread far within the chest.

> M1b means the cancer has spread to one place beyond the chest.

> M1c means the cancer has spread to more than one place beyond the chest.

Guide 6 N scores	
N0	The cancer has not spread to lymph nodes.
N1	The cancer has spread to lymph nodes in the lung.
N2	The cancer has spread to lymph nodes in one or both of these places: • In the middle of the chest next to the lung with cancer • Below the windpipe
N3	The cancer has spread to lymph nodes in one or more of these places: • In the middle of the chest near the other lung • In the other lung • Near the collarbone

Assigning a stage

Cancer stages consist of combinations of TNM scores based on prognosis. A prognosis is the likely outcome of the cancer. See Guide 7 for a list of TNM scores by cancer stage.

After your doctors determine the TNM scores, the cancer you have will be assigned a stage:

> **Stage 1** consists of subgroups stage 1A and 1B.

> **Stage 2** consists of subgroups stage 2A and 2B.

> **Stage 3** consists of subgroups stage 3A, 3B, and 3C.

> **Stage 4** consists of subgroups stage 4A and 4B.

For some people, cancer staging is done twice

The stage before treatment is called the clinical stage. It is noted with a lowercase "c." An example is cN0.

A second staging occurs after surgery. It is based on tests of tissue removed from the body. It is called the pathologic stage and is marked with a lowercase "p." An example is pN1.

Some cancers may not be correctly staged until after surgical treatment. For example, all the lymph nodes with cancer might not be found until surgery. On the other hand, some nodes thought to have cancer may be cancer-free.

Guide 7 Stages of lung cancer	
Cancer stage	**TNM scores**
1A	T1, N0, M0
1B	T2a, N0, M0
2A	T2b, N0, M0
2B	T3, N0, M0 T1, N1, M0 T2, N1, M0
3A	T3, N1, M0 T4, N0, M0 T4, N1, M0 T1, N2, M0 T2, N2, M0
3B	T3, N2, M0 T4, N2, M0 T1, N3, M0 T2, N3, M0
3C	T3, N3, M0 T4, N3, M0
4A	Any T, Any N, M1a Any T, Any N, M1b
4B	Any T, Any N, M1c

Additional staging tests

The clinical stage of lung cancer is first based on the initial tests listed in Chapter 2. Your doctor may order more staging tests to plan for treatment. The results of these tests may change the clinical stage.

Bronchoscopy

A bronchoscopy is a procedure that allows doctors to see inside of airways. It is also used to biopsy lung tissue and certain lymph nodes. NCCN experts recommend a bronchoscopy for clinical stages 1, 2, and 3A. A bronchoscopy is not needed for some stage 3B and 3C cancers. If you will have surgery, the bronchoscopy may be done right before the operation.

Mediastinal evaluation

The space between your lungs is called the mediastinum. This space has many lymph nodes. These nodes are more likely to have cancer when the lung tumor is larger and closer to this area. They can be seen using procedures called mediastinoscopy, mediastinotomy, and image-guided biopsies.

An evaluation of mediastinal nodes may not be needed for stage 1A. For clinical stage 1B, 2, and 3A, these nodes should be checked.

Scopes for lung cancer staging

It is very important for your doctors to know which lymph nodes have cancer. There are a few methods for examining or removing lymph nodes in the lungs and between the lungs. Bronchoscopy and mediastinoscopy are two of those methods.

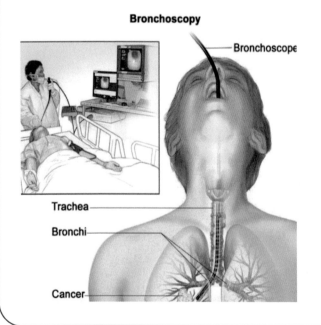

Bronchoscopy

Bronchoscope
Trachea
Bronchi
Cancer

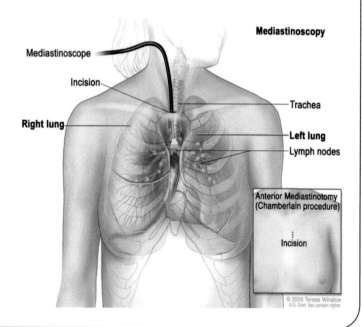

Mediastinoscopy

Mediastinoscope
Incision
Right lung
Trachea
Left lung
Lymph nodes
Anterior Mediastinotomy (Chamberlain procedure)
Incision

© 2006 Teresa Winslow
U.S. Govt. has certain rights

A mediastinal evaluation is not needed for all stage 3B and 3C cancers. Lymph nodes along the collarbone may be checked instead.

Brain MRI

Lung cancer tends to spread to the brain. Magnetic resonance imaging (MRI) may show small brain tumors that aren't causing symptoms. It uses a magnetic field and radio waves to make pictures. Contrast should be used.

MRI is not needed for clinical stage 1A but is an option for stage 1B. It is needed for clinical stage 2 and stage 3. If MRI can't be done, you may get computed tomography (CT) with contrast of your head.

MRI of spine and thoracic inlet

Some stage 2B and stage 3 lung cancers are superior sulcus tumors. This type of tumor starts at the top of the lung. It typically grows into the chest wall.

This tumor may have grown next to your spine, blood vessels, or nerves. In this case, MRI of your spine and thoracic inlet is needed. The thoracic inlet is the center of a ring of bones at the top of the ribcage.

Breathing tests

Treatment options depend on the clinical stage of the cancer. But, for some people, options are also based on how well their lungs work. There are three pulmonary function tests to assess how well you breathe:

> Spirometry involves blowing into a tube to measure how much air and how fast you breathe.

> A gas diffusion test involves breathing in a harmless gas and measuring how much you breathe out. It tells how much oxygen travels from your lungs into your blood.

> Body plethysmography involves sitting in a small room and breathing into a tube. This test measures how much air your lungs can hold and how much air is left in your lungs after you exhale.

People will ask how they can help. Be specific. For example, you could say, 'You can cook for me. Please pack meals in 4-ounce containers because that is all I can handle at any one time.'"

– Diane
Cancer survivor

Options for primary treatment

Not everyone with lung cancer receives the same treatment. Doctors plan treatment based on many factors, including:

> The cancer stage, which is explained earlier in this chapter

> The number of primary tumors

> Challenges to treating the cancer

> Your health

What is a primary tumor?
A primary tumor is the main mass of cancer cells in the lung. Two or more unrelated masses of cancer cells are called multiple primary tumors.

Most people with lung cancer have one primary tumor. People with one primary tumor can have separate yet related lung tumors. These separate tumors are sometimes called satellite tumors.

What is primary treatment?
Primary treatment is the main treatment used to rid your body of cancer. There are three types of primary treatment used for early and locally advanced lung cancers:

> **Surgery** is a treatment that removes tumors or organs with cancer.

> **Radiation therapy** most often uses high-energy x-rays to treat lung cancer.

> **Chemoradiation** is treatment with both chemotherapy and radiation therapy. Chemotherapy uses powerful drugs to kill cancer cells.

Options for primary treatment are based on the clinical stage of the cancer. See Guide 8 to learn which treatments may be options for you.

When possible, surgery is used for primary treatment. Your surgeon will assess if surgery is an option based on several factors:

> Can the tumor be fully removed from your body.

> Are you healthy enough to have lung cancer surgery.

More information on surgery is in Chapter 5. Learn about the types of surgery used to remove lung cancer and other types of treatments that you may receive.

What if surgery is not an option? In this case, treatment options are based on where the cancer is in the chest:

> Cancer that is only in the lung may be treated with radiation therapy. Read Chapter 6 for more information.

> When lung cancer is in and outside of the lung, chemoradiation is standard treatment. More information on chemoradiation is in Chapter 7.

Guide 8
Options for primary treatment of early and locally advanced lung cancers by stage

Stage	TNM score	Surgery	Radiation therapy	Chemoradiation
1A	T1, N0, M0	●	●	
1B	T2a, N0, M0	●	●	
2A	T2b, N0, M0	●	●	
2B	T3, N0, M0 (No invasive growth into nearby tissues)	●	●	
2B	T3, N0, M0 (Invasive growth) T1, N1, M0 T2, N1, M0	●		●
3A	T3, N1, M0 T4, N0, M0 T4, N1, M0 T1, N2, M0 T2, N2, M0	●		●
3B	T3, N2, M0 (No invasive growth into nearby tissues)	●		●
3B	T3, N2, M0 (Invasive growth) T4, N2, M0 T1, N3, M0 T2, N3, M0			●
3C	T3, N3, M0 T4, N3, M0			●

Clinical trials

Despite advances in treatment, more research is needed. Many lung cancers are not cured. Improving treatment is made possible with clinical trials.

A clinical trial is a type of medical research study. After being developed and tested in a laboratory, potential new ways of fighting cancer need to be studied in people. If found to be safe and effective in a clinical trial, a drug, device, or treatment approach may be approved by the U.S. Food and Drug Administration (FDA).

Everyone with cancer should carefully consider all of the treatment options available for their cancer type, including standard treatments and clinical trials. Talk to your doctor about whether a clinical trial may make sense for you.

Phases

Most cancer clinical trials focus on treatment. Treatment trials are done in phases.

> **Phase I trials** study the dose and safety of an investigational drug or treatment approach.

> **Phase II trials** study how well the drug or approach works against a specific type of cancer.

> **Phase III trials** test the drug or approach against a standard treatment. If the results are good, it may be approved by the FDA.

> **Phase IV trials** study the long-term safety and benefit of an FDA-approved treatment.

Who can enroll?

Every clinical trial has rules for joining, called eligibility criteria. The rules may be about age, cancer type and stage, treatment history, or general health. These requirements ensure that participants are alike in specific ways and that the trial is as safe as possible for the participants.

Informed consent

Clinical trials are managed by a group of experts called a research team. The research team will review the study with you in detail, including its purpose and the risks and benefits of joining. All of this information is also provided in an informed consent form. Read the form carefully and ask questions before signing it. Take time to discuss with family, friends, or others you trust. Keep in mind that you can leave and seek treatment outside of the clinical trial at any time.

Start the conversation

Don't wait for your doctor to bring up clinical trials. Start the conversation and learn about all of your treatment options. If you find a study that you may be eligible for, ask your treatment team if you meet the requirements. Try not to be discouraged if you cannot join. New clinical trials are always becoming available.

Frequently asked questions

There are many myths and misconceptions surrounding clinical trials. The possible benefits and risks are not well understood by many with cancer.

Will I get a placebo?

Placebos (inactive versions of real medicines) are almost never used alone in cancer clinical trials. It is common to receive either a placebo with a standard treatment or a new drug with a standard treatment. You will be informed, verbally and in writing, if a placebo is part of a clinical trial before you enroll.

Are clinical trials free?
There is no fee to enroll in a clinical trial. The study sponsor pays for research-related costs, including the study drug. You may, however, have costs indirectly related to the trial, such as the cost of transportation or child care due to extra appointments. During the trial, you will continue to receive standard cancer care. This care is billed to—and often covered by—insurance. You are responsible for copays and any costs for this care that are not covered by your insurance.

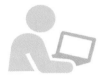

Finding a clinical trial

In the United States

NCCN Cancer Centers
NCCN.org/cancercenters

The National Cancer Institute (NCI)
cancer.gov/about-cancer/treatment/clinical-tri-als/search

Worldwide

The U.S. National Library of Medicine (NLM)
clinicaltrials.gov/

Need help finding a clinical trial?

NCI's Cancer Information Service (CIS)
1.800.4.CANCER (1.800.422.6237)
cancer.gov/contact

Key points

> A cancer stage is a rating of the growth and spread of cancer.

> A TNM system is used to score different areas of cancer growth.

> There are 4 main stages of lung cancer.

> For some people, cancer staging is done twice. The staging before treatment is called the clinical stage. The pathologic stage is based on test of tissue removed during surgery.

> Based on the cancer stage, you may get more tests. You may get more scans and procedures to get a more accurate cancer stage. You may get lung function tests to assess how well your lungs work.

> Doctors use the cancer stage to plan treatment. Surgery is a standard treatment for stage 1, 2, and 3 cancers. If surgery is not an option, radiation therapy or chemoradiation may be done instead.

> Clinical trials are a type of research. New ways of fighting cancer are studied among people in clinical trials. A clinical trial may be an option in addition to standard treatment.

5
Surgery

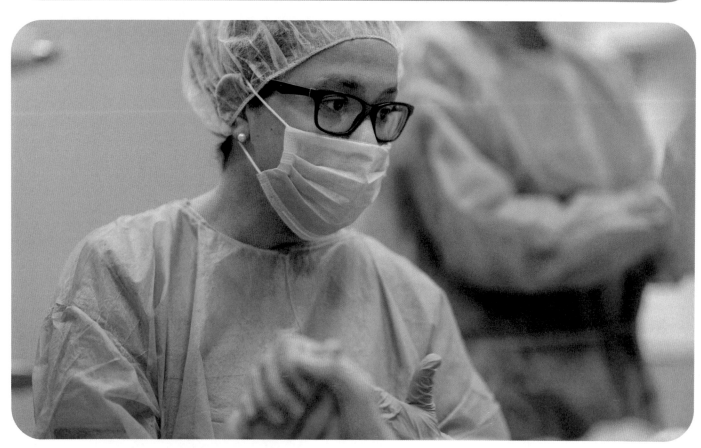

Surgery is a standard treatment for lung cancer, but the treatment approach differs between people. Read this chapter to learn how doctors tailor treatment for each person.

Types of surgery

The goal of surgery is to remove all of the cancer from the body. The tumor will be removed, along with some normal-looking tissue around its rim. The normal-looking tissue is called the surgical margin.

There are 5 types of lung surgery:

> Wedge resection removes a small part of a lobe.

> Segmentectomy removes a large part of a lobe.

> Lobectomy removes an entire lobe.

> Sleeve lobectomy removes an entire lobe and part of the main airway.

> Pneumonectomy removes an entire lung

Which surgery you will have depends on where the tumor has grown and how well your

Lung cancer surgery

There are 5 common lung cancer surgeries. The most common are lobectomy and pneumonectomy and are shown below. A sleeve lobectomy removes a lobe and part of the main airway called the bronchus. Wedge resection and segmentectomy remove only part of a lobe.

Lobectomy

Cancer

Lymph nodes

Lobe removed

© 2006 Terese Winslow
U.S. Govt. has certain rights

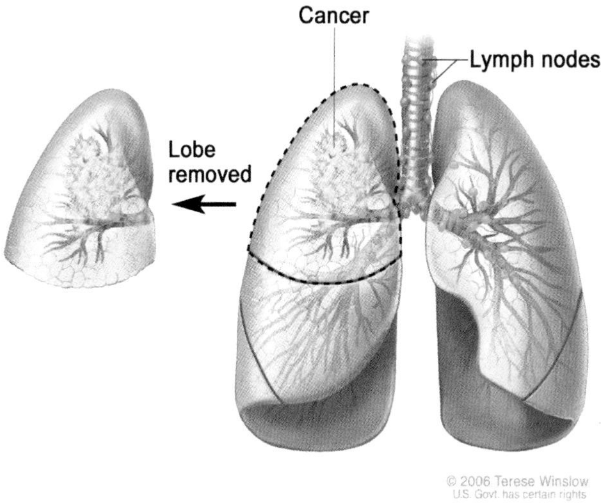

Pneumonectomy

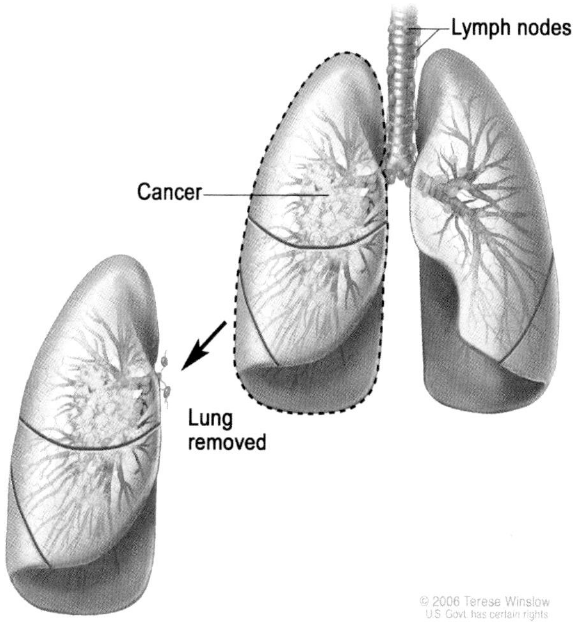

Lymph nodes

Cancer

Lung removed

© 2006 Terese Winslow
U.S. Govt. has certain rights

lungs work. The preferred surgery for most lung cancers is a lobectomy.

If T3 or T4 tumors are invasive, lung tissue as well as the invaded tissue will be removed together. The invaded tissue may include structures next to the lung, such as ribs and fat. This surgery is called an en-bloc resection.

Lymph node surgery

During surgery, lymph nodes that have or may have cancer will also be removed. To remove nodes, some organs may need to be moved or cut. There are two methods to remove lymph nodes.

- › A systematic lymph node sampling removes some nodes in the lung and between the lungs.

- › A lymph node dissection removes as many nodes as possible from the lung and between the lungs.

Surgical methods

Removal of a lung tumor can sometimes be done with one of two methods:

- › The classic method is thoracotomy. Tissue is removed through a large opening in the chest. Surgeons use a knife-like tool called a scalpel. Sometimes, part of the rib needs to be removed, too.

- › Thoracoscopy is a newer method. A small camera and surgical tools are inserted through small openings. Thoracoscopy can be done with or without help from a robot. It is also called video-assisted thoracoscopic surgery (VATS).

Treatments used with surgery

Most stage 1 cancers will be treated with only surgery. In contrast, it is rare for stage 2 and stage 3 lung cancers to be treated only with surgery. Instead, a combination of treatments is used to cure or control the cancer. See Guide 9 for a list of other treatments used with surgery.

Your treatment team will decide if other treatment is needed based on several factors:

- › If the tumor grew into nearby tissue

- › How likely the cancer will spread or come back after surgery

- › How helpful versus how harmful is the treatment

- › If the cancer cells have *EGFR* or PD-L1 biomarkers

Biomarker tests detect cell proteins that help the lung cancer grow. These tests may be done on a biopsy sample or the tissue removed during surgery.

Order of treatments

The order of treatments used with surgery differs between people. The order mainly depends on the cancer stage. There are two terms that convey the order of a treatment:

- › Induction therapy is the first treatment received

- › Adjuvant therapy follows surgery

The goal of induction therapy is to reduce the extent of cancer. It is sometimes given before surgery to make removal of the tumor easier. It may also relieve symptoms caused

Guide 9
Treatments used with surgery

Radiation therapy	Radiation therapy treats cancer in one area of the body with high-energy x-rays. It is sometimes used after surgery of early cancers.
Chemotherapy	Chemotherapy destroys fast-growing cells, including cancer cells, wherever they are in the body. It is given as a slow injection into a vein called an infusion. Either cisplatin or carboplatin is used with another type of chemotherapy.
Chemoradiation	Chemoradiation is treatment with both radiation therapy and chemotherapy. Sequential chemoradiation is the use of one treatment then the other. Concurrent chemoradiation is the use of both treatments at the same time.
Targeted therapy	Targeted therapy stops the specific ways by which cancer cells live, survive, and die. Osimertinib (Tagrisso) is a targeted therapy of lung cancers with abnormal genes called *EGFR exon 19* deletions and *EGFR L858R* mutations. It is a pill that can be taken at home and is started after chemotherapy is finished.
Immunotherapy	Immunotherapy is a treatment that engages your body's defense against disease—the immune system. Atezolizumab (Tecentriq) is an immunotherapy of lung cancers with a protein called PD-L1 on at least 1 percent of the cancer cells. It is started after chemotherapy is finished and is given by infusion.
Chemoimmunotherapy	Chemoimmunotherapy is treatment with both immunotherapy and chemotherapy. For lung cancer, an immunotherapy called nivolumab (Opdivo) is used. It is given by infusion.

by the cancer. Induction therapy may consist of chemotherapy with or without radiation or chemoimmunotherapy.

Adjuvant therapy is given after surgery to treat any cancer that may remain. Treatment is partly based on tests of the normal-looking tissue around the tumor, called the surgical margin.

Before surgery, your treatment team will know if you will likely receive adjuvant chemotherapy. If adjuvant therapy is likely, induction chemotherapy or chemoimmunotherapy may be an option instead.

Surgery by cancer stage

Your treatment team will plan treatment based on the cancer stage. More specifically, the plan is based on TNM scores described in Chapter 4. Your treatment team can show you which of the options below apply to you.

Stage 1A
Stage 1A cancer is very likely to be only in the lung. It is usually only treated with surgery.

Stage 1B
The growth of stage 1B cancer is very limited, so the cancer is often fully removed. Adjuvant chemotherapy is only received if the cancer is highly likely to return. Based on biomarker testing, osimertinib may be received as well.

Surgical margin

The tumor will be removed, along with some normal-looking tissue around its rim. The normal-looking tissue is called the surgical margin. The surgical margin will be tested for cancer. Adjuvant treatment is based on if there is cancer in the margins.

R0 margin No cancer in margin	**R1 margin** Cancer is found in margin with lab tests	**R2 margin** Cancer is easily seen in margin
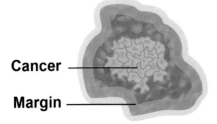	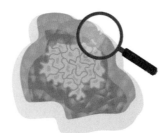	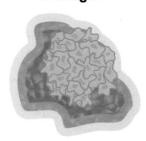

Cancer ——

Margin ——

Stage 2A

Treatment of stage 2A is almost the same as stage 1B. The difference is that atezolizumab is also an option for some stage 2A cancers after chemotherapy is completed.

Limited stage 2B and 3A

Some 2B and 3A cancers appear mainly confined to tissue inside the lung. Some may have grown into the main airway called the bronchus.

After surgery, chemotherapy is often used for adjuvant treatment. Based on biomarker testing, osimertinib or atezolizumab may be received as well. If cancer likely remains where the tumor was, chemoradiation may be used instead of chemotherapy.

Stage 2B and stage 3 with invasion and stage 3A with T4 tumors

Some stage 2B and stage 3 lung cancers are not confined to lung. A lung tumor may be scored T3 or T4 because it has grown into (invaded) nearby tissue, such as the chest wall or a blood vessel. Stage 3A also includes large T4 tumors that haven't invaded structures next to the lung.

Surgery is a common treatment if the cancer has not spread to lymph nodes (N0) or only to lymph nodes inside the lungs (N1).

The preferred treatment approach is to start with surgery. Chemotherapy is often used for adjuvant treatment, and based on biomarker testing, osimertinib or atezolizumab may be received as well. If cancer likely remains where the tumor was, chemoradiation may be used instead of chemotherapy.

Another approach is to start with concurrent chemoradiation or chemotherapy. Your surgeon may proceed with surgery if the tumor looks smaller on scans. A boost of radiation therapy may be received to treat any remaining cancer at the surgical site.

Stage 2B and stage 3 superior sulcus tumors with invasion

Superior sulcus tumors are a distinct subset of invasive lung cancers. They start at the top of the lung and typically grow into the chest wall.

Surgery is often an option for T3 tumors. The first treatment is chemoradiation followed by surgery.

Surgery is less likely an option for T4 tumors. Concurrent chemoradiation may shrink the tumor enough for surgery.

After surgery, chemotherapy is used for adjuvant treatment. Based on biomarker testing, osimertinib or atezolizumab may be received as well.

Stage 3A and 3B with N2 scores

Some stage 3 cancers have spread to N2 lymph nodes. N2 nodes are in the middle of the chest next to the lung with cancer. Some are right below the windpipe. Some of these cancers may be treated with surgery.

Induction chemotherapy with or without radiation may control the cancer growth. If it works, surgery may be an option. After surgery, you may get radiation therapy if you didn't have it before.

Side effects of surgery

All cancer treatments can cause unwanted health issues. Such health issues are called side effects. Some side effects may be harmful to your health. Others may just be unpleasant.

Side effects depend on many factors. These factors include the treatment type, length or dose of treatment, and the person.

Common side effects of any surgery are pain, swelling, and scars. Pain can be intense after lung surgery. Pain and swelling often fade away in the weeks after surgery.

Numbness near the surgical area may be long-lasting. There is a chance of infection, which may cause pneumonia. There's also a chance of a collapsed lung, which is called pneumothorax.

Many effects of treatment quickly resolve after treatment ends. Long-term effects start during treatment and persist after treatment is done. Less often, effects start long after treatment has ended.

Ask your treatment team for a complete list of side effects of your treatments. Also, tell your treatment team about any new or worse symptoms you get. There may be ways to help you feel better. There are also ways to prevent some side effects.

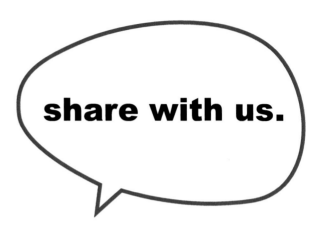

share with us.

Take our <u>survey</u>
And help make the
NCCN Guidelines for Patients
better for everyone!

NCCN.org/patients/comments

Key points

> Surgery is a common treatment of lung cancer. The goal is to remove the lung tumor and any lymph nodes with cancer.

> There are 5 types of lung surgery that range from removing a piece of a lobe to removing the entire lung.

> Other treatments are often used with surgery to treat lung cancer. They may be given before or after surgery.

> Treatment options largely depend on where the cancer has grown and spread.

> Early cancers are usually treated with surgery. If some cancer cells may remain, more treatment will be received after surgery.

> Advanced cancers are less likely to be treated with only surgery. Treatment is often given before surgery to stop the growth of the cancer. Surgery may follow if the first treatment has good results.

> Learn about the side effects of your treatments. Let your treatment team know about any new or worsening symptoms.

The good news is that today the medical industry has made great advances in treating cancer. They create a custom designed treatment specifically for you."

– Steve
   Cancer survivor

6
Radiation therapy

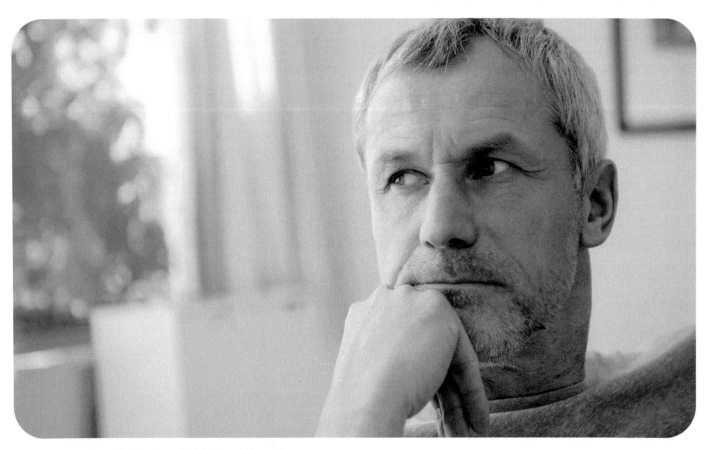

Radiation therapy is a common treatment of lung cancer. This chapter explains how radiation therapy treats lung cancer and some things to expect during treatment.

How radiation therapy is used

Radiation therapy uses high-energy x-rays or particles to treat lung cancer. It damages cancer cells. The cancer cells either die or stop making new cancer cells.

Radiation therapy is used in many ways to treat early and locally advanced lung cancers:

> Radiation therapy is sometimes received after surgery to treat any remaining cancer near to where the tumor was.

> Radiation therapy is sometimes combined with chemotherapy (chemoradiation) as described in Chapter 7.

> Radiation therapy may be the main (also called primary) treatment of stage 1 and some stage 2 lung cancers. The goal is to cure the cancer. Doctors refer to this treatment as definitive radiation therapy.

A radiation oncologist is a doctor who is an expert in treating cancer with radiation. This doctor will lead a team that designs your treatment plan and provides treatment.

Types of radiation therapy

External beam radiation therapy (EBRT) is the most common method used for lung cancer. A large machine makes radiation beams that are shaped to the form of the tumor. The highest radiation dose is aimed at the cancer. A much lower dose is given to nearby tissue.

There are several common techniques of EBRT:

> **Intensity-modulated radiation therapy (IMRT)** delivers x-ray beams that very closely match the shape of the target and spare more normal tissue. Treatment is finished in about 6 weeks.

> **Three-dimensional conformal radiation therapy (3D-CRT)** delivers an x-ray beam that matches the shape of the target but may not be as focused as IMRT. Treatment is finished in about 6 weeks.

> **Stereotactic ablative radiotherapy (SABR)** treats cancer with very precise, high-dose x-ray beams. It delivers a very high dose of radiation per treatment, but for only a few treatments. Treatment is finished in 1 to 1½ weeks.

> **Proton therapy** treats cancer with proton beams. Proton beams deliver radiation mostly within the tumor. Treatment is completed in about 6 weeks.

Radiation therapy is typically delivered daily from Monday through Friday. Treatment visits are about 15 minutes. Some radiation oncologists deliver SABR treatment 2 to 3 times per week.

Curing lung cancer with radiation

EBRT is used when trying to cure lung cancer. Any of the techniques described before may be used though NCCN experts prefer SABR. SABR has been shown to work well. It controls cancer growth and extends life.

Overcoming treatment challenges

A lung tumor is harder to target than some other tumors in the body. To account for these challenges, advanced methods may be used:

> Four-dimensional computed tomography (4D-CT) may be used for treatment planning. It's like a movie of your lungs moving.

> Positron emission tomography with computed tomography (PET/CT) may be used to know where to deliver the radiation treatment.

> Motion control methods may be used to keep you still during treatment.

Treatment after radiation therapy

For stage 1B or stage 2 cancer, you may get chemotherapy after radiation. Chemotherapy can treat cancer cells that radiation did not. Large tumors and very abnormal-looking cancer cells may have spread to places outside the radiation field.

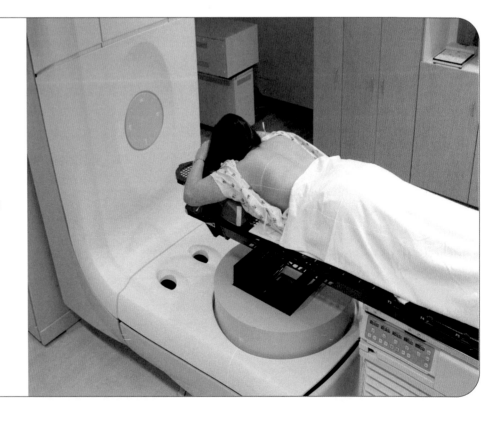

Radiation therapy

Radiation therapy is often delivered from a large machine. The x-rays or particles pass through skin and travel to the tumor. Healthy tissue is protected using modern types of treatment.

Side effects of radiation

Radiation therapy does not:

> Cause pain during a treatment session—people feel nothing at all

> Make you radioactive

On the other hand, radiation therapy may cause health problems called side effects. Side effects of radiation therapy are cumulative. This means they build up slowly and are worse at the end of treatment.

> Fatigue and skin changes are common. Often, people describe skin changes as like a sunburn.

> Near the end of treatment, you may have pain when swallowing.

> Although not common, your lung may become inflamed over the months of treatment. This can cause sudden shortness of breath or cough. Call your radiation oncologist immediately if you have these symptoms.

Ask your treatment team for a complete list of side effects of your treatments. Also, tell your treatment team about any new or worse symptoms you get. There may be ways to help you feel better. There are also ways to prevent some side effects.

Key points

> Radiation therapy uses high-energy x-rays or particles to treat lung cancer.

> There are several ways radiation therapy is used to treat lung cancer. When used to cure cancer, it is called definitive radiation therapy.

> Radiation therapy is most often delivered from outside the body using a large machine.

> Several techniques are available to cure lung cancer. Stereotactic ablative radiotherapy (SABR) has very good results.

> You may receive chemotherapy after radiation therapy.

> After several treatment sessions, you may feel fatigued and your skin sunburned.

7
Chemoradiation

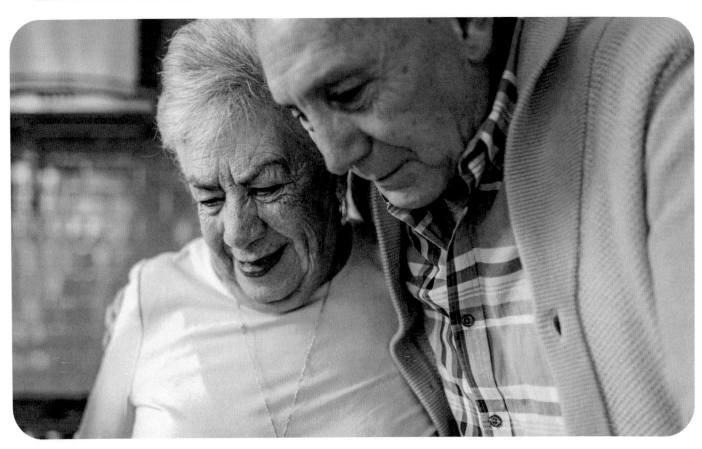

Chemoradiation uses the power of two treatments. Read this chapter to learn the options and what to expect.

How chemoradiation is used

Chemoradiation is a combination of these two treatments:

> Chemotherapy – It stops the process by which cells make more cells, so it affects fast-growing cells like cancer.

> Radiation therapy – It uses high-energy x-rays or particles to damage cancer cells. The cancer cells either die or can't make more cancer cells.

Chemoradiation is used in two ways to treat early and locally advanced lung cancers:

> Chemoradiation is sometimes part of surgical treatment as described in Chapter 5.

> Chemoradiation may also be the main (also called primary) treatment of lung cancer. When the goal is to cure the cancer, it is called definitive chemoradiation.

Types of chemotherapy

Radiation therapy is described in Chapter 6. The types of radiation therapy and what to expect are explained. Here's a short description of chemotherapy.

Chemotherapy is a type of medication. It is prescribed by doctors called medical oncologists. Medical oncologists know which medications treat which cancers.

For early and locally advanced lung cancer, more than one type of chemotherapy is received. Often, cisplatin or carboplatin—drugs made with platinum—is used with another drug for treatment. These regimens are called platinum-doublet chemotherapy.

You will not receive chemotherapy every day. Instead, it is given in cycles of treatment days followed by days of rest. Giving chemotherapy in cycles gives your body a chance to recover after receiving chemotherapy.

You will need to go to a treatment center to get chemotherapy. The chemotherapy will be slowly injected into your vein. This is called an infusion. The drugs travel in your bloodstream to treat cancer throughout your body.

Curing lung cancer with chemoradiation

Definitive chemoradiation is a treatment option for some stage 2B and stage 3 lung cancers. There are two scheduling approaches to delivering chemoradiation:

> Concurrent chemoradiation means that chemotherapy and radiation therapy are given at the same time. This schedule is followed when surgery is not an option.

> Sequential chemoradiation means you will first complete chemotherapy then receive radiation therapy. This schedule may be followed if concurrent treatment may be too harmful for you.

Chemoradiation differs between people

Your treatment team will make a plan for you based on several factors, such as:

> Concurrent or sequential schedule

> Type of lung cancer

> How well a chemotherapy works (preferred regimens work well and are safe)

Chemotherapy cycles vary in length depending on which drugs are used. Ask your doctor how many cycles you will have and how many days of treatment there are within a cycle. A list of recommended regimens is in Guide 10.

Radiation therapy also differs between people based on treatment schedule:

> For concurrent chemoradiation, radiation therapy is typically delivered in 30 to 35 small doses called fractions over 6 to 7 weeks.

> For sequential chemoradiation, you may be treated with about 15 higher-dose fractions.

Guide 10
Chemotherapy regimens for chemoradiation

Concurrent chemoradiation	For adenocarcinoma, large cell, and rare types of lung cancers: • Carboplatin, pemetrexed (preferred) • Cisplatin, pemetrexed (preferred) • Carboplatin, paclitaxel (preferred) • Cisplatin, etoposide (preferred) For squamous cell carcinomas: • Carboplatin, paclitaxel (preferred) • Cisplatin, etoposide (preferred)
Sequential chemoradiation	For adenocarcinoma, large cell, and rare types of lung cancers: • Cisplatin, pemetrexed (preferred) For squamous cell carcinomas: • Cisplatin, gemcitabine (preferred) • Cisplatin, docetaxel (preferred) For any type of lung cancer: • Cisplatin, vinorelbine • Cisplatin, etoposide • Carboplatin, paclitaxel (sometimes useful) • Carboplatin, gemcitabine (sometimes useful) • Carboplatin, pemetrexed (sometimes useful)

Consolidation treatment

The goals of consolidation are to bolster the results of treatment and to delay the cancer from coming back. Durvalumab (Imfinzi) is used as consolidation treatment after definitive chemoradiation.

Durvalumab is a type of immunotherapy called a checkpoint inhibitor. Immunotherapy uses the immune system to kill cancer cells. Durvalumab works by enabling T cells to attack cancer cells.

Durvalumab is slowly injected into a vein (infusion). It may take 60 minutes to get the full dose. Infusions are received every 2 or 4 weeks for 1 year.

Side effects of treatment

Side effects are unwanted health problems caused by treatment. All cancer treatments cause side effects. But, side effects differ between people based on the type and length of treatment as well as the person.

Side effects from chemotherapy are caused by the death of fast-growing normal cells. You may feel nauseated during treatment. You may lose your hair. Side effects are typically worse with concurrent chemoradiation compared with sequential chemoradiation.

Immune checkpoint inhibitors can cause your immune cells to attack healthy cells in your body. Read about immune-related side effects in *NCCN Guidelines for Patients: Immunotherapy Side Effects, Immune Checkpoint Inhibitors* at NCCN.org/patientguidelines.

Ask your treatment team for a complete list of side effects of your treatments. Also, tell your treatment team about any new or worse symptoms you get. There may be ways to help you feel better. There are also ways to prevent some side effects.

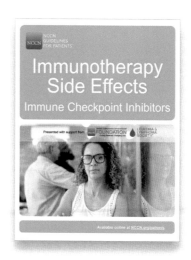

Key points

> Chemoradiation is a treatment with both chemotherapy and radiation therapy. It may be used to try to cure lung cancer.

> Chemotherapy for lung cancer often consists of a drug made with platinum and one other drug. It is slowly infused into a vein.

> Often, chemotherapy and radiation therapy are given at the same time.

> Durvalumab may be received after chemoradiation to delay the return of cancer.

> Let your treatment team know about any new or worsening symptoms.

8
Survivorship care

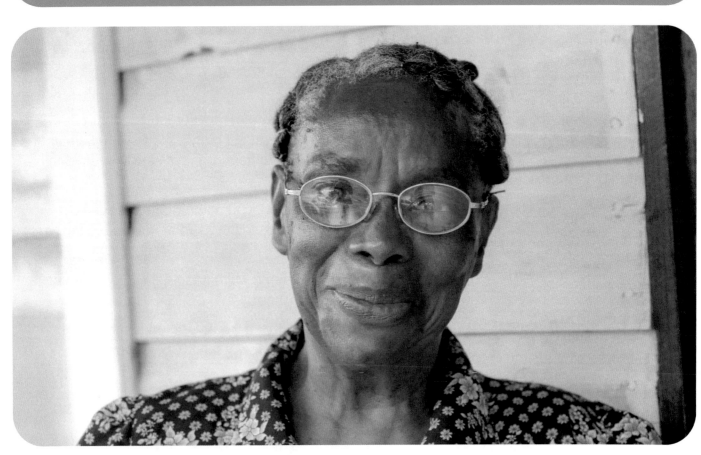

Survivorship care includes recovering from cancer and promoting health. This chapter reviews a few key parts of survivorship care.

Cancer tests

While lung cancer can sometimes be cured, it is very important to monitor for the return of the cancer. The return of cancer is called a recurrence. It is also important to be checked for other types of cancer.

Surveillance

Survivorship care should include a schedule of tests for recurrence. Routine testing for cancer recurrence is called surveillance. Surveillance is started when there are no signs of cancer after treatment. Early detection of a recurrence will allow for timely treatment. See Guide 11 for a schedule of tests.

You may be at risk for a second lung cancer. Anyone who has been treated and cured of one lung cancer is at risk for getting a new lung cancer. Your risk increases as you age. If you smoke, your chance for cancer increases the longer you smoke.

Guide 11 Surveillance	
Your treatment did not include radiation therapy	Every 6 months for 2 to 3 years: • Medical history • Physical exam • CT of the chest with or without contrast If test results are normal, then repeat every year: • Medical history • Physical exam • Low-dose CT
Your treatment did include radiation therapy	Every 3 to 6 months for 3 years: • Medical history • Physical exam • CT of the chest with or without contrast If normal results, then repeat every 6 months for 2 years: • Medical history • Physical exam • Low-dose CT If test results are normal, then repeat every year: • Medical history • Physical exam • Low-dose CT

Cancer screening

A second cancer is a possible late effect of some cancer treatments. Ask your doctor about your risk for another cancer. If you have a high risk for certain cancers, you may enroll in a screening program. Cancer screening is routine testing for cancer before cancer symptoms start. Not every type of cancer has a screening program, though.

There are cancer screening programs for:

> Prostate cancer

> Breast or cervical cancer

> Colorectal cancer

> Skin cancer

Managing side effects

All cancer treatments can cause health issues called side effects. Many effects of treatment quickly resolve after treatment ends. An example is nausea and vomiting. Long-term effects start during treatment and persist after treatment is done. Less often, effects start long after treatment has ended. These are called late effects.

During health visits, your health care providers will assess for side effects. They will provide treatment for side effects as needed. Read about common effects in *NCCN Guidelines for Patients: Survivorship Care for Cancer-Related Late and Long-Term Effects*, available at NCCN.org/patientguidelines.

Learning to manage side effects is well worth the effort!

– Jon
  Lung cancer survivor

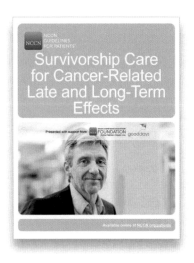

Survivorship Care for Cancer-Related Late and Long-Term Effects

Disease prevention

Another part of follow-up care is to prevent diseases. Such care can include getting immunization shots for the flu, herpes, shingles, and other diseases. Dental cleaning and exams on a regular basis can prevent disease, too.

It's important to start or keep a healthy lifestyle. Healthy living may improve your health and well-being. It may also help prevent the cancer from returning. Work with your treatment team to set goals and make plans for healthy living.

Common goals for healthy living include:

> Seeing a primary care provider on a regular basis

> Being physically active and avoiding inactivity

> Eating healthful foods

> Limiting or avoiding drinking alcohol

> Achieving and maintaining a healthy body weight

> Not using tobacco

> Avoiding infections

> Getting safe vaccines

Read about preventing poor health in *NCCN Guidelines for Patients: Survivorship Care for Healthy Living*, available at NCCN.org/patientguidelines.

Key points

> Your cancer doctors will monitor for a return of lung cancer. Early detection will allow for timely treatment. You will also be checked for other cancers, including a second lung cancer. If you have a high risk for certain cancers, you may enroll in a screening program.

> Some side effects of treatment are long-term or may appear years later. At follow-up visits, your doctor will assess for side effects. Tell your doctor about any new or worse symptoms. There may be ways to prevent or treat side effects.

> Preventing diseases is a part of follow-up care. Such care can include getting immunization shots and dental cleaning. Healthy living may improve your health and prevent disease.

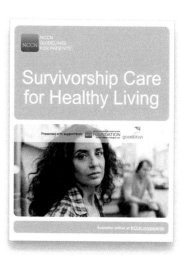

9
Making treatment decisions

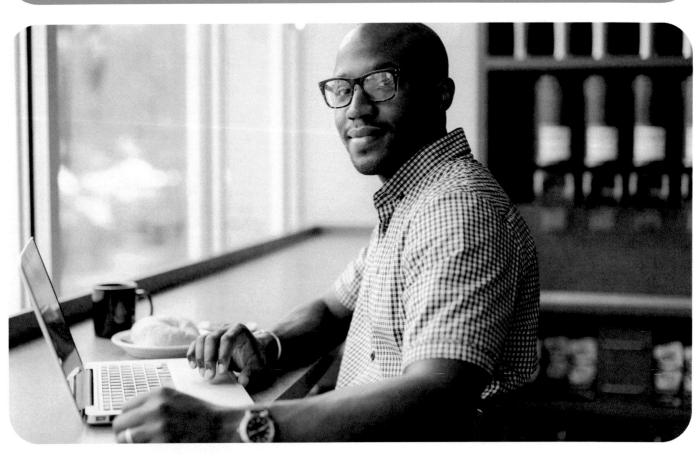

It's important to be comfortable with the cancer treatment you choose. This choice starts with having an open and honest conversation with your doctors.

It's your choice

In shared decision-making, you and your doctors share information, discuss the options, and agree on a treatment plan. It starts with an open and honest conversation between you and your doctor.

Treatment decisions are very personal. What is important to you may not be important to someone else. Some things that may play a role in your decisions:

> What you want and how that might differ from what others want

> Your religious and spiritual beliefs

> Your feelings about certain treatments like surgery or chemotherapy

> Your feelings about pain or side effects such as nausea and vomiting

> Cost of treatment, travel to treatment centers, and time away from work

> Quality of life and length of life

> How active you are and the activities that are important to you

Think about what you want from treatment. Discuss openly the risks and benefits of specific treatments and procedures. Weigh options and share concerns with your doctor. If you take the time to build a relationship with your doctor, it will help you feel supported when considering options and making treatment decisions.

Second opinion
It is normal to want to start treatment as soon as possible. While cancer can't be ignored, there is time to have another doctor review your test results and suggest a treatment plan. This is called getting a second opinion, and it's a normal part of cancer care. Even doctors get second opinions!

Things you can do to prepare:

> Check with your insurance company about its rules on second opinions. There may be out-of-pocket costs to see doctors who are not part of your insurance plan.

> Make plans to have copies of all your records and imaging studies sent to the doctor you will see for your second opinion. Images can be burned onto a CD.

Support groups
Many people diagnosed with cancer find support groups to be helpful. Support groups often include people at different stages of treatment. Some people may be newly diagnosed, while others may be finished with treatment. If your hospital or community doesn't have support groups for people with cancer, check out the websites listed in this book.

Questions to ask

Possible questions to ask your doctors are listed on the following pages. Feel free to use these questions or come up with your own. Be clear about your goals for treatment and find out what to expect from treatment.

Questions to ask about testing and staging

1. What tests will I have?

2. Do I need a biopsy? What kind of biopsy do I need? Will enough tissue be removed for future testing? What are the risks?

3. How do I prepare for testing?

4. What if I am pregnant?

5. Where do I go to get tested? How long will the tests take and will any test hurt?

6. Should I bring someone with me? Should I bring a list of my medications?

7. How soon will I know the results and who will explain them to me?

8. Would you give me a copy of the pathology report and other test results?

9. What type of lung cancer do I have? What is the stage? Has the cancer spread far?

10. Can this cancer be cured? If not, how well can treatment stop the cancer from growing?

11. Who will talk with me about the next steps? When?

Questions to ask about treatment options

1. What are my treatment options? Are you suggesting options other than what NCCN recommends? If yes, why?

2. Do your suggested options include clinical trials? Please explain why.

3. What will happen if I do nothing?

4. How do my age, overall health, and other factors affect my options? What if I am pregnant or planning to get pregnant?

5. Does any option offer a cure or long-term cancer control? Are my chances any better for one option than another? Less time-consuming? Less expensive?

6. How do you know if treatment is working? How will I know if treatment is working?

7. What are my options if treatment stops working?

8. What are the possible complications? What are the short- and long-term side effects of treatment?

9. What can be done to prevent or relieve the side effects of treatment?

10. What supportive care services are available to me during and after treatment?

11. Can I stop treatment at any time? What will happen if I stop treatment?

Questions to ask about clinical trials

1. Are there clinical trials for my type of cancer?

2. What are the treatments used in the clinical trial?

3. What does the treatment do?

4. Has the treatment been used before? Has it been used for other types of cancer?

5. What are the risks and benefits of this treatment?

6. What side effects should I expect? How will the side effects be controlled?

7. How long will I be in the clinical trial?

8. Will I be able to get other treatment if this doesn't work?

9. How will you know the treatment is working?

10. Will the clinical trial cost me anything? If so, how much?

Questions to ask about getting treated

1. Will I have to go to the hospital or elsewhere? How often? How long is each visit?

2. What do I need to think about if I will travel for treatment?

3. Do I have a choice of when to begin treatment? Can I choose the days and times of treatment?

4. How do I prepare for treatment? Do I have to stop taking any of my medicines? Are there foods I will have to avoid?

5. Should I bring someone with me when I get treated?

6. Will the treatment hurt?

7. What should I do if a side effect gets bad when my cancer center is closed?

8. How much will the treatment cost me? What does my insurance cover?

9. Will I miss work or school? Will I be able to drive?

10. Is home care after treatment needed? If yes, what type?

11. How soon will I be able to manage my own health?

12. When will I be able to return to my normal activities?

Resources

American Cancer Society
cancer.org/cancer/lung-cancer.html

American Lung Association
lung.org

American Lung Cancer Screening Initiative
alcsi.org

Caring Ambassadors Program, Inc.
lungcancercap.org

Free ME from Lung Cancer
freeMEfromLungCancer.org

GO2 Foundation for Lung Cancer
go2foundation.org

Lung Cancer Alliance
lungcanceralliance.org

Lung Cancer Research Foundation
lcrf.org

LUNGevity Foundation
LUNGevity.org

National Cancer Institute (NCI)
cancer.gov/types/lung

National Coalition for Cancer Survivorship
canceradvocacy.org/toolbox

NCCN Patient Resources
NCCN.org/patients

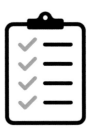

We want your feedback!

Our goal is to provide helpful and easy-to-understand information on cancer.

Take our survey to let us know what we got right and what we could do better:

NCCN.org/patients/feedback

Words to know

ablation
A treatment that destroys very small tumors with heat or cold.

adenocarcinoma
A cancer of cells that line organs and make fluids or hormones.

adjuvant treatment
Treatment that is given to lower the chances of the cancer returning.

AJCC
American Joint Committee on Cancer

alveoli
The tiny sacs in the lungs where gases are transferred in and out of the blood.

biopsy
A procedure that removes fluid or tissue samples to be tested for a disease.

board certified
A status for doctors who finished training and passed exams in a specialized field of medicine.

body plethysmograph
A test of how much air is in your lungs after inhaling or exhaling.

bronchioli
Small airways within the lungs.

bronchoscope
A device that is guided down the throat to work inside the airways.

bronchoscopy
A procedure to work inside the airways with a device that is guided down the throat.

bronchus
One of the two main airways that extends into the lungs.

cancer screening
Routine testing for cancer in people without symptoms.

cancer stage
A rating of the outlook of a cancer based on its growth and spread.

carcinoma
A cancer of cells that line the inner or outer surfaces of the body.

chemistry profile
A lab test of the amount of 8 chemicals in a sample of blood. Also called metabolic panel.

chemoradiation
A cancer treatment with both cell-killing drugs and high-energy rays.

chemotherapy
Cancer drugs that stop the cell life cycle so cells don't increase in number.

chest wall
The layer of muscle, bone, and fat that protects the vital organs.

chronic obstructive pulmonary disease (COPD)
Lung damage or too much mucus that makes breathing hard.

clinical stage
The rating of the extent of cancer before treatment is started.

clinical trial
A type of research that assesses how well health tests or treatments work in people.

complete blood count (CBC)
A lab test that measures the parts of the blood.

computed tomography (CT)
A test that uses x-rays from many angles to make a picture of the insides of the body.

contrast
A dye put into your body to make clearer pictures during imaging.

CRX
chest x-ray

diagnosis
An identification of an illness based on tests.

endobronchial ultrasound–guided transbronchial needle aspiration (EBUS-TBNA)
A procedure that removes lung tissue with a needle on an imaging device guided down the windpipe.

endoscopic ultrasound–guided fine-needle aspiration (EUS-FNA)
A procedure that removes fluid with a needle on an imaging device guided through a natural opening.

esophagus
The tube-shaped organ between the mouth and stomach.

external beam radiation therapy (EBRT)
Radiation therapy received from a machine outside the body.

FDG
fluorodeoxyglucose

gas diffusion
A test that uses harmless gas to measure how much you breathe out.

GGN
ground-glass nodule

GGO
ground-glass opacity

immunotherapy
A treatment with drugs that help the body find and destroy cancer cells.

intensity-modulated radiation therapy (IMRT)
Treatment with radiation that uses small beams of different strengths.

invasion
The growth of cancer from where it started into another tissue.

large-cell lung carcinoma
A cancer of lung cells that lack features to classify as another type of lung cancer.

lobe
A clearly seen division in an organ.

lobectomy
An operation that removes a whole lobe of an organ.

low-dose computed tomography (LDCT)
A test that uses small amounts of radiation to make pictures of the insides of the body.

lymph node
A small, bean-shaped, disease-fighting structure.

magnetic resonance imaging (MRI)
A test that uses radio waves and powerful magnets to make pictures of the insides of the body.

mediastinoscope
A device that is guided through a small cut to do work inside the chest.

mediastinoscopy
A procedure to do work in the chest with a device passed through a small cut in the skin.

mediastinum
The area of the chest between the lungs.

medical history
A report of all your health events and medications.

metastasis
The spread of cancer from the first tumor to a new site.

multiple primary tumor
One or more unrelated masses of cancer cells.

navigational bronchoscopy
A procedure to do work in the smallest airways with a device guided down the windpipe.

NCCN
National Comprehensive Cancer Network

nodule
A small mass of tissue.

non-small cell lung cancer (NSCLC)
A cancer that starts in lung cells that are not small.

non-solid nodule
A small tissue mass of low density.

part-solid nodule
A small tissue mass with areas of low and high density.

pathologic stage
A rating of the extent of cancer based on tests given after treatment.

pathologist
A doctor who's an expert in testing cells to find disease.

physical exam
A review of the body by a health expert for signs of disease.

pneumonectomy
An operation that removes the entire lung.

positron emission tomography (PET)
A test that uses radioactive material to see the shape and function of body parts.

positron emission tomography/computed tomography (PET/CT)
A test that uses two picture-making methods to show the shape and function of tissue.

primary tumor
The main mass of a certain type of cancer cells.

prognosis
The likely course and outcome of a disease based on tests.

proton therapy
Radiation therapy that uses protons to treat a disease. Also called hadron therapy.

pulmonary function tests
A set of breathing tests to test the strength of the lungs.

pulmonologist
A doctor who's an expert in lung diseases.

radial endobronchial ultrasound (EBUS) bronchoscopy
A procedure to do work inside the lung with an imaging device guided down the windpipe.

radiation oncologist
A doctor who's an expert in treating cancer with radiation.

radiation therapy
A treatment that uses intense energy to kill cancer cells.

respiratory system
The group of organs that transfers gases in and out of the body.

risk factor
Anything that increases the chance of an event.

segmentectomy
An operation that removes a large part of a lobe.

side effect
An unhealthy or unpleasant physical or emotional response to treatment.

sleeve lobectomy
An operation to remove an entire lobe and part of the bronchus.

small cell lung cancer (SCLC)
A cancer of small lung cells.

solid nodule
A small mass of tissue of high density.

spirometry
A test that uses a tube to measure how fast you breathe.

squamous cell carcinoma
A type of cancer of thin and flat cells that line the surface of organs.

stereotactic ablative radiotherapy (SABR)
Treatment with high-dose radiation within one or a few sessions. Also called SBRT.

superior sulcus tumor
A mass of cancer cells that starts at the top of the lung and easily grows into the chest wall.

supportive care
Health care that includes symptom relief but not cancer treatment. Also sometimes called palliative care.

surgery
An operation to remove or repair a part of the body.

surgical margin
The normal-looking tissue around a tumor that was removed during an operation.

thoracic radiologist
A doctor who's an expert in reading imaging tests of the chest.

thoracic surgeon
A doctor who's an expert in operating on organs inside the chest.

thoracoscopy
A procedure to do work in the chest with a device passed through a small cut in the skin. Also called VATS.

three-dimensional conformal radiation therapy (3D-CRT)
A treatment with radiation that uses beams matched to the shape of the tumor.

trachea
The airway between the throat and airway into the lungs. Also called the windpipe.

transthoracic needle biopsy (TTNB)
A procedure that removes tissue samples with a thin needle guided through the ribs.

ultrasound
A test that uses sound waves to take pictures of the inside of the body.

video-assisted thoracic surgery (VATS)
A procedure to do work in the chest with a device passed through a small cut in the skin. Also called thoracoscopy.

wedge resection
An operation that removes a small part of a lobe.

NCCN Contributors

This patient guide is based on the NCCN Clinical Practice Guidelines in Oncology (NCCN Guidelines®) for Non-Small Cell Lung Cancer, Version 3.2022. It was adapted, reviewed, and published with help from the following people:

Dorothy A. Shead, MS
Senior Director
Patient Information Operations

Laura J. Hanisch, PsyD
Patient Information Program Manager

Susan Kidney
Senior Graphic Design Specialist

The NCCN Clinical Practice Guidelines in Oncology (NCCN Guidelines®) for Non-Small Cell Lung Cancer, Version 3.2022 were developed by the following NCCN Panel Members:

David S. Ettinger, MD/Chair
The Sidney Kimmel Comprehensive Cancer Center at Johns Hopkins

*Douglas E. Wood, MD/Vice Chair
Fred Hutchinson Cancer Research Center/ Seattle Cancer Care Alliance

Dara L. Aisner, MD, PhD
University of Colorado Cancer Center

Wallace Akerley, MD
Huntsman Cancer Institute at the University of Utah

Jessica R. Bauman, MD
Fox Chase Cancer Center

Ankit Bharat, MD
Robert H. Lurie Comprehensive Cancer Center of Northwestern University

Debora S. Bruno, MD, MS
Case Comprehensive Cancer Center/ University Hospitals Seidman Cancer Center and Cleveland Clinic Taussig Cancer Institute

Joe Y. Chang, MD, PhD
The University of Texas MD Anderson Cancer Center

Lucian R. Chirieac, MD
Dana-Farber/Brigham and Women's Cancer Center

Thomas A. D'Amico, MD
Duke Cancer Institute

Malcolm DeCamp, MD
University of Wisconsin Carbone Cancer Center

Thomas J. Dilling, MD, MS
Moffitt Cancer Center

Jonathan Dowell, MD
UT Southwestern Simmons Comprehensive Cancer Center

Scott Gettinger, MD
Yale Cancer Center/Smilow Cancer Hospital

Travis E. Grotz, MD
Mayo Clinic Cancer Center

Matthew A. Gubens, MD, MS
UCSF Helen Diller Family Comprehensive Cancer Center

Aparna Hegde, MD
O'Neal Comprehensive Cancer Center at UAB

Rudy P. Lackner, MD
Fred & Pamela Buffett Cancer Center

Michael Lanuti, MD
Massachusetts General Hospital Cancer Center

Jules Lin, MD
University of Michigan Rogel Cancer Center

Billy W. Loo, Jr., MD, PhD
Stanford Cancer Institute

Christine M. Lovly, MD, PhD
Vanderbilt-Ingram Cancer Center

Fabien Maldonado, MD
Vanderbilt-Ingram Cancer Center

Erminia Massarelli, MD, PhD, MS
City of Hope National Medical Center

Daniel Morgensztern, MD
Siteman Cancer Center at Barnes-Jewish Hospital and Washington University School of Medicine

Thomas Ng, MD
The University of Tennessee Health Science Center

Gregory A. Otterson, MD
The Ohio State University Comprehensive Cancer Center - James Cancer Hospital and Solove Research Institute

Jose M. Pacheco, MD
University of Colorado Cancer Center

Sandip P. Patel, MD
UC San Diego Moores Cancer Center

Gregory J. Riely, MD, PhD
Memorial Sloan Kettering Cancer Center

Jonathan Riess, MD
UC Davis Comprehensive Cancer Center

Steven E. Schild, MD
Mayo Clinic Cancer Center

Theresa A. Shapiro, MD, PhD
The Sidney Kimmel Comprehensive Cancer Center at Johns Hopkins

Aditi P. Singh, MD
Abramson Cancer Center at the University of Pennsylvania

James Stevenson, MD
Case Comprehensive Cancer Center/ University Hospitals Seidman Cancer Center and Cleveland Clinic Taussig Cancer Institute

Alda Tam, MD
The University of Texas MD Anderson Cancer Center

Tawee Tanvetyanon, MD, MPH
Moffitt Cancer Center

Jane Yanagawa, MD
UCLA Jonsson Comprehensive Cancer Center

Stephen C. Yang, MD
The Sidney Kimmel Comprehensive Cancer Center at Johns Hopkins

Edwin Yau, MD, PhD
Roswell Park Comprehensive Cancer Center

NCCN Staff

Kristina Gregory, RN, MSN, OCN
Vice President, Clinical Information Programs

Miranda Hughes, PhD
Oncology Scientist,/Seniior Medical Writer

* Reviewed this patient guide. For disclosures, visit NCCN.org/disclosures.

NCCN Cancer Centers

Abramson Cancer Center
at the University of Pennsylvania
Philadelphia, Pennsylvania
800.789.7366 • pennmedicine.org/cancer

Case Comprehensive Cancer Center/
University Hospitals Seidman Cancer
Center and Cleveland Clinic Taussig
Cancer Institute
Cleveland, Ohio
800.641.2422 • UH Seidman Cancer Center
uhhospitals.org/services/cancer-services
866.223.8100 • CC Taussig Cancer Institute
my.clevelandclinic.org/departments/cancer
216.844.8797 • Case CCC
case.edu/cancer

City of Hope National Medical Center
Los Angeles, California
800.826.4673 • cityofhope.org

Dana-Farber/Brigham and Women's
Cancer Center | Massachusetts General
Hospital Cancer Center
Boston, Massachusetts
617.732.5500 • youhaveus.org
617.726.5130
massgeneral.org/cancer-center

Duke Cancer Institute
Durham, North Carolina
888.275.3853 • dukecancerinstitute.org

Fox Chase Cancer Center
Philadelphia, Pennsylvania
888.369.2427 • foxchase.org

Fred & Pamela Buffett Cancer Center
Omaha, Nebraska
402.559.5600 • unmc.edu/cancercenter

Fred Hutchinson Cancer
Research Center/Seattle
Cancer Care Alliance
Seattle, Washington
206.606.7222 • seattlecca.org
206.667.5000 • fredhutch.org

Huntsman Cancer Institute
at the University of Utah
Salt Lake City, Utah
800.824.2073 • huntsmancancer.org

Indiana University
Melvin and Bren Simon
Comprehensive Cancer Center
Indianapolis, Indiana
888.600.4822 • www.cancer.iu.edu

Mayo Clinic Cancer Center
Phoenix/Scottsdale, Arizona
Jacksonville, Florida
Rochester, Minnesota
480.301.8000 • Arizona
904.953.0853 • Florida
507.538.3270 • Minnesota
mayoclinic.org/cancercenter

Memorial Sloan Kettering
Cancer Center
New York, New York
800.525.2225 • mskcc.org

Moffitt Cancer Center
Tampa, Florida
888.663.3488 • moffitt.org

O'Neal Comprehensive
Cancer Center at UAB
Birmingham, Alabama
800.822.0933 • uab.edu/onealcancercenter

Robert H. Lurie Comprehensive Cancer
Center of Northwestern University
Chicago, Illinois
866.587.4322 • cancer.northwestern.edu

Roswell Park Comprehensive
Cancer Center
Buffalo, New York
877.275.7724 • roswellpark.org

Siteman Cancer Center at Barnes-
Jewish Hospital and Washington
University School of Medicine
St. Louis, Missouri
800.600.3606 • siteman.wustl.edu

St. Jude Children's
Research Hospital/
The University of Tennessee
Health Science Center
Memphis, Tennessee
866.278.5833 • stjude.org
901.448.5500 • uthsc.edu

Stanford Cancer Institute
Stanford, California
877.668.7535 • cancer.stanford.edu

The Ohio State University
Comprehensive Cancer Center -
James Cancer Hospital and
Solove Research Institute
Columbus, Ohio
800.293.5066 • cancer.osu.edu

The Sidney Kimmel Comprehensive
Cancer Center at Johns Hopkins
Baltimore, Maryland
410.955.8964
www.hopkinskimmelcancercenter.org

The University of Texas
MD Anderson Cancer Center
Houston, Texas
844.269.5922 • mdanderson.org

UC Davis
Comprehensive Cancer Center
Sacramento, California
916.734.5959 • 800.770.9261
health.ucdavis.edu/cancer

UC San Diego Moores Cancer Center
La Jolla, California
858.822.6100 • cancer.ucsd.edu

UCLA Jonsson
Comprehensive Cancer Center
Los Angeles, California
310.825.5268 • cancer.ucla.edu

UCSF Helen Diller Family
Comprehensive Cancer Center
San Francisco, California
800.689.8273 • cancer.ucsf.edu

University of Colorado Cancer Center
Aurora, Colorado
720.848.0300 • coloradocancercenter.org

University of Michigan
Rogel Cancer Center
Ann Arbor, Michigan
800.865.1125 • rogelcancercenter.org

University of Wisconsin
Carbone Cancer Center
Madison, Wisconsin
608.265.1700 • uwhealth.org/cancer

UT Southwestern Simmons
Comprehensive Cancer Center
Dallas, Texas
214.648.3111 • utsouthwestern.edu/simmons

Vanderbilt-Ingram Cancer Center
Nashville, Tennessee
877.936.8422 • vicc.org

Yale Cancer Center/
Smilow Cancer Hospital
New Haven, Connecticut
855.4.SMILOW • yalecancercenter.org

Index

Made in the USA
Middletown, DE
26 July 2023

35764589R00040